GIFT

FROM MY SON

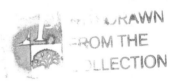

GIFT
FROM MY SON

Autism Redefined

Keli Lindelien

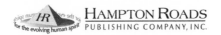

HAMPTON ROADS
PUBLISHING COMPANY, INC.

Excerpt from *Joy's Way* by Brugh Joy, copyright © 1979 by Brugh Joy. Used
by permission of Jeremy P. Tarcher, an imprint of Penguin Group (USA) Inc.

Excerpts from *Nobody Nowhere* by Donna Williams, copyright © 1992 by
Donna Williams. Used by permission of Times Books,
a division of Random House, Inc.

Excerpts from *What Your Doctor May Not Tell You About Children's
Vaccinations* by Stephanie Cave, M.D. Copyright © 2001
by Stephanie Cave, M.D. By permission of Warner Books, Inc.

Cover design by Marjoram Productions
Cover photography © 2004 Laurents Hamels/Photo Alto/Picture Quest

Hampton Roads Publishing Company, Inc.
1125 Stoney Ridge Road
Charlottesville, VA 22902

434-296-2772
fax: 434-296-5096
e-mail: hrpc@hrpub.com
www.hrpub.com

If you are unable to order this book from your local bookseller,
you may order directly from the publisher.
Call 1-800-766-8009, toll-free.

Library of Congress Cataloging-in-Publication Data
Lindelien, Keli.
 Gift from my son : autism redefined / Keli Lindelien.
    p. cm.
 Includes bibliographical references.
 ISBN 1-57174-391-X (5 1/2 x 8 1/2 tp : alk. paper)
 1. Lindelien, Benjamin--Health. 2. Autistic children--United
States--Biography. 3. Autism in children--Alternative treatment. I. Title.
 RJ506.A9L54 2004
 362.198'9285882'0092--dc22
                                        2004001562

10 9 8 7 6 5 4 3 2 1
Printed on acid-free paper in Canada

Dedication

To Dave for his absolute and enduring love
and support during this time,

To Karis, for her selfless love and compassion,
and for teaching me about the things I couldn't see,

To Benjamin, who had the most difficult job of all.

Contents

Foreword

Autism affects children with all kinds of different personalities, from all sorts of backgrounds. They can share a label and even many of the external behaviors used by professionals to diagnose the condition, and yet have very different underlying causes involved in their condition, some known, some still being discovered.

Some people with autism have a strong family history of autism-associated conditions. In addition, or even underlying their autism, some have severely disabling neurotransmitter imbalances associated with other conditions such as bipolar "disorder," obsessive-compulsive "disorder," or Tourette's syndrome. Professionals are now discovering that for this particular group, these conditions can begin in infancy and in severe and disabling cases are sometimes manageable through a combination of nutritional measures and appropriate, "safer," very low doses of conventional medicine without deadifying the personhood of the patient.

Some people with autism develop severe gut and immune system disorders, and epilepsy is also very common. These may underlie information processing and developmental and behavioral differences, and have sometimes been found to respond well to interventions in the fields of nutritional and complementary medicine.

Some people with autism have severe and disabling chronic fight-flight responses, which I call Exposure Anxiety, sometimes for no other reason than that the neurotransmitter responsible for this state is out of balance.

Some people with autism have environmental illnesses brought on by exposure to environmental toxins and may be relatively treatable with some forms of complementary medicine.

Some people with autism have left-right hemisphere integration problems and many may be stuck in a predominantly right-brain reality where sensing dominates and interpretive thinking is difficult to grasp, let alone master. Two of the main therapies currently used for this group include chiropractic and patterning techniques sometimes referred to as "Brain Gym."

Where the left-brain dominant person with Asperger's may find it hard to turn off their interpretive mind, the right-brain dominant person with autism may be relatively "mindless" yet so highly sensing as to be overwhelmed by involuntarily merging with the pattern, theme, and feel of everyone and everything around them. At the same time, the person with autism may be unable to connect well enough via the more mind-driven world of surface-level, verbal, wordy communication to communicate this and be surrounded by those who do not use his or her system. Just as the incredible interpretive mind of the person with Asperger's can leave us in awe and we have come to acknowledge its usefulness in society, Keli Lindelien's work challenges that there is no reason why we should not equally celebrate the exceptional sensate we might find at the autistic end of the spectrum.

Ben is not every autistic child—for there is no such poster child. But his journey awakens us to the importance of understanding an aspect of autism so challenging to the predominantly scientific and analytical minds of most professionals in the field of autism: sensing.

Keli Lindelien is a person who understood something of the world of sensing and lost touch with it, then revisited it through her son, Ben. A well-known and highly sensing autistic person named Jim Sinclair once summarized that parents faced with a child with autism can mourn or they can embrace the adventure ahead of them. Going out on a limb in ways the analytical skeptic may never dare, Keli Lindelien found her own way to embrace that adventure. However questionable anyone may find her unique experiences or theories, they would struggle to criticize the honor of her motives. She did not seek to "normalize" her son out of fear of being sentenced to life with "an autistic," but rather used his condition as a tool for her own self-discovery, believing that her son could reach his potential through acceptance and respect for his way of navigating in the world. She didn't seek to give him her bridge but to provide him with the tools with which to build his own, not as a means for him to lose his autistic world, but with a view to finding the shared places between two worlds.

—*Donna Williams, autistic artist and author of* Nobody
Nowhere *and seven other books in the field of autism,*
www.donnawilliams.net

Acknowledgments

I wish to express my deepest gratitude to the following people who contributed to our understanding of Benjamin and the writing of this book:

My dear friend Ron Bryan, for providing inspiration and tireless physics explanations and editing assistance, and for his serendipitous introduction to my publisher.

Betty and Bob Unterberger, for their loving support during my journey of discovery, for teaching me the value of meditation, and for their editing expertise.

My long-time ally, Debra Ellis, who first gave enthusiastic support for my writing.

Pat Cleere, for her friendship, creative insight, and suggestions, and for introducing me to the idea that my thoughts create.

Rob Robb, for giving us the courage to change our lives.

Rabyn Judith Pillsbury, for her intuitive insight, support, and suggestions about the role of altered states of awareness and for the use of her beautiful poem, *Whispers*.

My mother and Ed and my father and Anne, for all their support and assistance on this journey.

Sean Harribance, for his friendship and support.

Donna Williams, for providing a precious glimpse into her

world, for her courage, and for her review and editing advice on the autism material in the manuscript.

Behice Kutay, David Malin, Susan Hartzog, Melody Hart, and Liz Parker, for their role in increasing Benjamin's comfort level—I cannot thank them enough.

Brandi Maler, Mary Forrest, and Geana Bassham, for their patience, determination, and loving encouragement.

Janet Boutton, Miroslava Lopez, Elvia Soto, and Norma Fischer, Benjamin's classroom teachers in Texas, and Kathi Harris, Betty Coopersmith, Nola Falcocchia, and Martha Tejera, his teachers in California, for their faith in Benjamin, and for their kindness.

Judith Wells-Walberg, Berkeley Soukup, Anne Wehrly, Susan Leonard, Kelle Wood, and Susan Catlett, for their assistance and support in Benjamin's educational experiences.

Laurie Monroe and The Monroe Institute, for providing a refuge for discovery.

Sarah Hilfer, for her assistance with the manuscript and Anne Louque, for the cover design.

And finally, to my publisher and editor, Frank DeMarco, for his friendship and strong encouragement to write this book "for the parents of autistic children."

A Parent's Tears

A life more than lonely,
A soul more than empty,
A heart that is only
The place where you hold
The love and the moments
Your mind has forgotten
From days not remembered
And stories untold.
If I could remember
The secrets once whispered
And promises made
Long before I was born,
Then I'd know the reason
For what life has shown me
For all that I praise
And for all that I mourn.
For each day we live
There are questions unanswered
And answers unquestioned,
Far worse, I suppose,
Oh, what shall become of
The words never spoken,
The tears never shed
And thoughts no one else knows.

—*Author unknown*[1]

Introduction

This is not a story about a magic bullet. This is a story about acceptance—and love. This is the story of a child whose differences have been staggering at times. It is about the child who rocked my world. His condition would cause me to question all of my beliefs about conventional medicine, about life after death, about traditional values, about God, and about myself. I have been compelled to scrutinize every facet of my life and the meaning of my existence in the past several years. This is a story about change and about hope.

A month before Benjamin was born, I began my early morning meditation. Due to the size of my enormous belly, I was finding it difficult to get into a relaxed state. As I closed my eyes following three or four attempts to find a comfortable position, I suddenly found myself in a white, ethereal place. I was sitting at the feet of a beautiful, loving being. I remember feeling love like I had never felt in my entire life. It permeated every cell and pore of my body and formed my very being. Tears flowed down my cheeks from the overwhelming joy I felt in his presence. Taking my face in his hands as I sat fascinated by the glimmering, yet translucent, sleeve of his robe, he asked, "Don't you know that I have been with you always?" His face was the most beautiful one I had ever seen, not because of its physical characteristics, but because of the powerful, all-encompassing love that emanated from him and enveloped me.

In this cosmic consciousness experience, I saw the God I had felt watching over me since I was a child. Recognizing the voice that I had heard many times in my early life, I once again remembered that he was real, tangible, and he loved and accepted my entire being. All the fragments of life's existence seemed to merge into a tapestry of light and color and splendor. I asked him what I should call him.

He replied, "If you must call me by a name, you may call me The Master."

I knew that I had never been alone. I had no idea at the time why it was imperative for me to be reminded of this fact.

In our culture, we are inundated with the idea that everyone should be the same, with the level of left-brain intelligence being our only guide to a person's worth and value to society. Material achievement is thought to be the primary goal. When you are in a position of "sameness," everything seems logical, rational, and safe. I believed that I was happy and secure with a life plotted out exactly as I had planned. My husband and I were highly educated. He earned a master's degree in engineering when my daughter was a baby, and I held a law degree. I loved my job, where I met interesting, exciting, and powerful people. I adored my charming, mild-mannered husband, and our beautiful daughter was an easy child. She was quick-witted and verbal and had inherited her father's charm. I thought I loved my life. When Benjamin entered our world, I was 36 years old.

I dreamed of attending my children's graduations and celebrating their marriages. I possessed all of the things that I had been told all my life would bring me happiness. I believed that I had the perfect life, doing all the things that I thought that I was supposed to do. I had carefully suppressed and ignored the emptiness and the longing for something more, for the meaningfulness of life itself.

My favorite university professor, Dr. Elizabeth Harper Neeld, in *A Sacred Primer: The Essential Guide to Quiet Time and Prayer*, quotes Clarissa Pinkola Estes's description of a little girl in a fairy tale whose red shoes would never stop dancing. I didn't realize it at the time, but I was that little girl:

> [T]he shoes danced the girl, rather than the other way around. . . . So dance and dance and dance she did. Over the highest hills and through the valleys, in the rain and the

snow and in the sunlight, she danced. She danced in the darkest night and through sunrise and she was still dancing at twilight. But it was not good dancing. It was terrible dancing, and there was no rest for her.[2]

When I was face to face with Benjamin's condition, I found myself tumbling in a sea of uncertainty, not sure what to do next. I was in a situation that I could not escape. Before, when something was uncomfortable, I could move, change jobs, change friends, or simply push it out of my life. I could just keep dancing. Now, I had nowhere to run and no place to hide. I had to stop dancing for the child who needed me, and no one else was up to the task. The responsibility of that alone was terrifying. Then add the pity, the disapproval, the second-guessing, and the well-meaning suggestions of others who had never been faced with the inescapable situation of a special-needs child, and the world suddenly seemed formidable. At the end of the day, I was the one who had to get it done, to hold it all together. Although my husband was very supportive, I was the one who had to step up when the resources were exhausted. I was at the end of the line with one crisp buck in my hand. What if I didn't have the fortitude? What if I just decided one day that I couldn't handle it anymore. How could I live with myself if I ever got to that point? Thank you, Benjamin, for showing me my fear.

Special-needs children reveal to us our deepest fears. They show us our fear of being different, of being dependent on another, of not being perfect. As a child, I spent enormous amounts of time molding myself into whoever everyone else wanted me to be. I always knew that there was something different about me, something bubbling just below the surface that I could not name. At 13 years old, I sat across from my grandmother one evening as she sat on our daybed. As I rocked in our rocker, I realized that it was the last time that I was going to see her in this life. As I studied her thin frame, her pale, almost translucent skin, and her silver hair, I was undisturbed by this revelation, as it came with a sense of peace and calmness that I had never experienced in my teenage life. I spent the next few minutes silently memorizing her face, watching her mannerisms, studying the lines in her hands, and feeling my love for her. As I hugged and kissed her that evening, I absorbed her essence, knowing that it would have to last. I was emotionally prepared when my mother came into my room the next morning and told me that she had passed over quietly in her sleep.

One of my mother's greatest gifts to me was her acknowledgment of my "knowings." She always treated my premonitions with respect, as if they were the product of countless hours of diligent effort. She often said that she would like to take me somewhere to be studied, in order to find out more about why I knew the things I knew. There just never was enough time or money. Other pressing matters always intervened.

My mother's respect for these "knowings" increased when I announced one day that I had an extreme dislike of one of her friends.

"Why don't you like her?" she asked.

"I don't know, there is just something about her that I don't like. I don't trust her. I don't know why," I responded.

The woman had been hired by my mother's friend to perform bookkeeping duties for his small business. My mother was influential in helping her land the job. The woman subsequently embezzled almost ten thousand dollars from the man. My mother told me that she would never doubt my intuition again.

(My mother was no stranger to these feelings herself. A lump was discovered in my mother's lung, and she was admitted to M. D. Anderson Cancer Center in Houston for a biopsy. As she lay in bed the morning before the surgery, she felt herself become engulfed in a beautiful white light. The light washed over her, entering at the top of her head and exiting at her feet. The light bathed her with a sense of peace, unlike any sensation that she had felt before. She knew that she had been healed. Shortly before the surgery, the surgeon decided to take another chest X-ray for further study. The X-ray revealed that the lump had disappeared, and only a small scar remained. Completely puzzled, the surgeon explained that it was as if the tumor had been burned away.)

At 16 years old, I discovered that letting others know of my abilities wasn't always safe. One day, the familiar awareness came over me. This time, I knew that my boyfriend's best friend was going to die. Two weeks later, he was murdered as I watched. We were in a grocery store parking lot that served as a weekend gathering spot for local high school kids. In the evenings, teenagers cruised up and down Tenth Street in their cars, stopping to talk and gathering in the parking lot. Probably 50 or 60 people stood in the parking lot that evening. Suddenly, I saw my boyfriend's best friend in what appeared to be a fight with another man. Everything transpired in slow motion. I was vaguely aware of my boyfriend struggling with another man. I couldn't breathe, and I couldn't move. It seemed as if time had simultaneously stopped and started to go backward. My awareness shifted as I watched from above as two men exchanged punches in one area, and two other men fought for control of a tire tool. I wasn't even aware that the man struggling for control of the tire tool was my boyfriend. It was just a strange, surreal movie being played out before me as I watched, unemotional and disassociated from any outcome.

My awareness suddenly shifted, settling back into my body with a thump. My boyfriend's best friend was lying in a pool of blood, moaning, and moving only slightly. "Call an ambulance," someone screamed. My boyfriend appeared beside me. He looked shaken. The ambulance came and the attendants quickly loaded up our friend. Someone threw our friend's cowboy hat into the ambulance, as if he would be looking for it. My boyfriend took my arm and led me to my car. We went to find the victim's wife, who just two weeks before had married our friend in a small ceremony at the local Baptist church. We found her at home and quickly made our way to the hospital, chatting and pretending that everything would be all right and our lives wouldn't be blown to pieces in the intervening hours.

As we walked into the hospital, she was told that her husband of two weeks had died of multiple stab wounds on his way to the hospital. I can still hear her screams ringing in my ears. I can still feel her fingers pressing into my back, holding on to me as if her grasping could somehow bring him back. Believing that a slight twist of fate could have placed me in her shoes with the love of *my* young life lying dead under the hospital drape, the curtain of childhood innocence fell heavily at my feet.

I suffered from extreme guilt for not warning our friend, for not doing something to prevent his death. This time, I told someone about my premonition. Upon discovering that I had foreseen this young man's death, I was accused by a member of the victim's fundamentalist Christian family of being "of the devil." This was extremely upsetting to me, since I had been raised in a fundamentalist Christian tradition. That same day, I had just concluded two days of testimony during which I endured relentless cross-examination, trying to help convict his killer. Although there were many people present, I was the only person who could identify one of the men. In a moment of calm detachment as the scene unfolded before me, the man who had struggled with my boyfriend turned and looked directly at me, his tortured face permanently etched in my psyche.

I suffered along with the victim's family. I agonized over whether my premonition had somehow caused his demise. I felt like a freak. I didn't know why I knew this or how. I did know that this ability set me apart, made me different. Suddenly, it was all about who would live and who would die. I simply shut it off and pushed it out of my life. It was easier to forget it than to deal with it. The price had just become too high.

Now, I found myself with an autistic child, whose hand flapping and unintelligible utterances could not be ignored. I was face to face with different, and he was a part of me, the part of me that I had carefully and methodically sealed up and separated from myself.

PART I

The Boy

1 The Arrival

We don't see things as they are. We see them as we are.

—the Talmud

Benjamin was so wanted, so desired. Because my life had been filled with girls, from the moment I thought about having a child, I always imagined having a son. My second pregnancy was uneventful. I was busy with my two-year-old daughter, Karis, our recently completed dream home, and my job. When I was newly pregnant, I asked Karis if the baby we were expecting would be a boy or a girl. She replied without hesitation, "a boy," and never changed her preference to have a brother.

Karis's name literally means "gift of grace." She has been one of the greatest gifts that my husband and I could have asked for and the greatest help to us on our journey with Benjamin. She adores him. I believe even then that she foresaw the tiny baby changing everything that we knew for certain to be real, the boy who would lead us from Texas to California, then to Australia, from conventional medicine to natural medicine, from ordinary values to values of the heart. She has always been a very wise child.

I started attending meditation classes the month that Benjamin was conceived and began communicating with him in my daily meditation. It began as a one-way conversation as I would tell him how much he was wanted and how everything would be all right. Before long, I seemed to be able to sense a communication coming back to me. It was as if he were reassuring me that everything would be all right. I was not even plagued with gestational diabetes as I had been during my first pregnancy. In the third month of my pregnancy, I asked in my meditation what Benjamin's life purpose would be. I received a straightforward answer: to be loved, to feel secure, and to learn compassion.

Due to my age, my obstetrician mentioned that I could undergo an amniocentesis to determine if there were any detectable problems with the baby. Not being the type of person who likes surprises, I was leaning toward doing the test so that I could either be sure that everything was fine or be prepared in case it was not. My husband wasn't in favor of doing the procedure, since there were risks to the baby. I was going back and forth in my mind about whether to do the procedure, not making much progress in making a decision.

One morning, as I was taking my shower, I suddenly felt the following words come into my awareness: "Why do you need a test for that which you already know?" I was shocked by the intensity of the words as they were perceived in my mind. I knew that the words weren't just mind chatter, since the words felt as if they were forced into my brain, rather than being produced by it, and the words were structured in a way that I would never speak. I would never have used those words to convey that information. After this incident, I was totally at peace with the decision to forego the procedure. I recognized the familiar "knowing" from my childhood but wondered why it had returned so abruptly, nearly 20 years after that fateful night when I watched a friend die.

When Benjamin was born, it was a relief, but it was not the emotional high that I had felt with my first child. I felt somewhat guilty about his birth seeming so uneventful, until they brought him to me early the next morning. As I looked at him, I suddenly felt an incredible and overwhelming sense of love and connection to him. As I held him up, looking directly into his pale blue eyes, the words "I have waited so long to see you" came from my lips, and I began to cry. Somehow, even then, I knew that I wasn't referring to the nine months that I had carried him. As our soul connection locked into place, the winds of change began to blow, slowly breathing life into unknown possibilities.

Benjamin was a beautiful blond-headed boy with piercing almond-shaped blue eyes, who reflected his father's Norwegian heritage. He was wide-eyed, good natured, and happy. As my husband is the only boy, he is the sole heir to the Lindelien name. He was the only grandson on my side of the family. He was our first son, and our last child. We all celebrated his birth.

When he was just a few weeks old, his grandmother told me that he had eyes that "looked all the way into your soul." Consistently taller and bigger than his peers, he was strikingly beautiful. My best friend commented that he was "the most beautiful baby she had ever laid eyes on." Even as a small child, he had his father's athletic build.

In the beginning, he seemed fairly normal, except for a severe allergy to milk, a small eczema patch on his face, and a rather extreme sensitivity to medications. I didn't think his sensitivity to medications was unusual, since my mother and I are both very sensitive to prescription drugs. Benjamin laughed, smiled, clapped his hands, and displayed behavior that seemed no different from my daughter's during her first few months of life.

When Benjamin was eight months old, he crawled into the base of our brick fireplace, gashing his left eyebrow. Blood poured down his face, but he didn't cry. Seeing the depth of the wound, I scooped him up, shouting to my daughter that we had to go to the doctor.

As we drove to the doctor's office, my daughter, sensing my distress, said, "Don't worry, Momma. Mrs. Rather is with us. Ben's going to be okay." She indicated that Mrs. Rather was sitting in the passenger seat of our van, watching over us.

I thanked Karis for her assurances and thanked Mrs. Rather for her timely appearance. Since Karis had been able to speak, Mrs. Rather had been her constant companion. When asked why she called her Mrs. Rather, she replied, "She told me that was her name." Karis pronounced her name "Rat-ter" with the emphasis on the last syllable.

We thought this was curious, since we didn't know anyone by this name. We referred to this woman as her imaginary friend until the day I saw Karis comparing the size of her foot to Mrs. Rather's. When I asked Karis what she looked like, she described an older woman in period clothing. I didn't fully understand what she was seeing at the time, but given my own experience with the unexplained, I didn't feel that I should discourage it.

After our arrival at the doctor's office, the pediatrician determined that stitches weren't necessary, but he would need to apply dermabond, a solution similar to household superglue, to hold the wound together so that it could heal. As the pediatrician called in his nurse to help hold Benjamin, he explained that we would have to hold Benjamin very tightly, as it was essential that he remain still, since the substance was to be applied very close to his eye. As his pediatrician leaned over to apply the substance, Benjamin followed his movements with his eyes. As the doctor applied the solution, he studied the doctor's face, without flinching or moving a muscle. The doctor commented, "I feel as though I'm treating a prizefighter." Even at this young age, he seemed to have an unusually high pain tolerance, or he understood exactly what was happening.

Benjamin spoke his first few words before he was a year old. He became very excited in certain situations, but his hand flapping and cooing were endearing. In some ways it was charming to see a child who could get so excited over the small things in life, such as the swirling of water going down the drain or the excitement of feeling the wind in his face. Sometimes, he would laugh and coo, interacting with someone, which wasn't unusual for a child, except that his attention wasn't focused on me, but on something just over my shoulder. Often, when he was alone in his bedroom, we heard him laughing and giggling, just like he did when we were playing with him. He walked at 13 months old.

At Benjamin's one-year checkup, I dutifully filled out the doctor's forms. He's right on target, I thought to myself. The appointment went quickly. The nurse came in to conclude the visit by giving his scheduled immunizations, the measles, mumps, and rubella (MMR) vaccine and the Varicella (chicken pox) vaccine. Benjamin was also given a blood test, to check the severity of his milk allergy. My heart went out to him being stuck twice with a needle and having so much blood drawn.

As we were leaving, I stopped at the front desk to handle the paperwork. The nurse practitioner happened by. I was on the board of directors of a child advocacy center, and she was the wonderful soul who performed all of the examinations on the sexually abused children who were referred to the center. As we chatted, Benjamin started fussing. We ignored his fussing, talking a little louder and faster. His discomfort escalating, Benjamin suddenly screamed out, "LET'S GO!" Our conversation stopped in mid-sentence.

"How old is that baby?" the receptionist behind the counter asked.

"He'll be one next week," I replied.

"Wow, smart one," she countered.

As I loaded Benjamin into our van, I noticed that his body was shaking slightly. The shaking was periodic, rather than constant, and appeared similar to a person's bodily sensation when exposed to something very distasteful, almost like a shudder. At the time I thought it was because he had gotten so upset in his doctor's office. Benjamin continued experiencing body "shudders" for the next several weeks.

Upon arriving home, I proudly recorded "said two words correctly" in his baby book. It would be more than two years before I could make that claim again.

At 18 months old, I looked into our backyard to see him walking down the slide on his play set. With his arms extended like a tightrope walker's, he carefully and easily made his way down the four-foot-tall slide to safety. He did this often, and never fell even once.

On one occasion, Benjamin was running in the park. A bee flew by and landed on his hand. As I ran over to swat at the bee, it flew away. I raised Ben's hand and could see the bee's stinger protruding slightly above his knuckle. I flicked the stinger out of his skin, taking care not to squeeze it but could see that his skin was already beginning to react to the sting. He vocalized a few sounds, waved his hand around a few times, then went back to playing. Wow, what a pain tolerance, I thought. I had no idea at that time that a high pain tolerance could be indicative of autism.

At his second birthday party, we invited a small group of children and several close relatives. When it was time to open his gifts, his sister and I performed the task, since he refused even to stay in the same room. He completely ignored us, running around the house, then jumping up and down on his trampoline positioned in front of the television. The birthday cake and candles remained unnoticed. He sat dully in his high chair, digging his fingers into the piece of cake I placed in front of him, staring off into nowhere. As far as Benjamin was concerned, the other people and children didn't even exist. He's just an unusually active little boy who isn't interested in anything that isn't physical, we told ourselves. The dark circles creeping in around his eyes should have told us otherwise.

We first began to realize that he was becoming very difficult to care for when he was almost two years old. I quit my job, telling my friends and family that Benjamin just seemed to need me more than my daughter had. He seemed to tantrum frequently and my mother was having a hard time dealing with him when I was working. He seemed to focus on certain things and it was almost impossible for him to switch from one activity to another. By the time he was two and a half years old, his day consisted of the following activities:

• Running for hours in wide circles while looking sideways

• Jumping up and down on a small trampoline while watching one of a handful of videos

• Eating a diet of beans, fruits, vegetables, bread, and french fries

• Sleeping (intermittently)

Like a small plastic windup toy, when he ran, Benjamin would go and go and go, as if he had been wound too tightly. He tried to expend all his excess energy at once. The problem was that something just kept winding him up. Once, he ran nonstop in wide circles in our backyard for over three hours. He never looked forward when he ran. He stared sideways, off into the distance. Aware of the images scooting by, he was unable to focus on them. If he were not allowed to do his chosen activity, he would throw himself on the floor, crying, kicking, and screaming. I had the bruises up and down my legs to prove it.

Even while watching his favorite videos, he was unable to be still. He jumped on his small trampoline, never looking down, never falling, his gaze locked on the television, sweat dripping from his face on hot Texas days. He communicated with me by crying, fussing, screaming, grunting, or occasionally pulling at me to lead me to a desired object. His verbal communication consisted of a variety of consonant and vowel sounds that tended to be repetitive and somewhat nonintentional. Occasionally an appropriate word would pop out of his mouth, usually only once, never to be repeated.

One day shortly before his diagnosis, I decided to try finger painting with Benjamin, since it had been one of his sister's favorite activities when she was his age. I sat him down at the plastic-covered kitchen table, carefully placing several opened jars of finger paint in front of him. He looked at the paint, then just sat there.

"Come on, Ben, put your fingers in it like this," I said.

I dipped the fingers of one of his hands in the paint. He whined and quickly rubbed the paint off onto the paper. I grabbed a spatula and ran it through the paint.

"Look, Benjamin, look at the designs," I prodded.

He stared blankly off into the distance. Where are you, Benjamin, I wondered. Sometimes it's like he doesn't even know I'm here, I thought. I snapped a photo of his first attempt at painting, then cleaned him up and put all the painting equipment away, trying to ignore the sinking feeling in the pit of my stomach.

Attempts to read to him met with the same fate. He simply wasn't interested, or couldn't focus on what I was saying. He couldn't sit still to listen to a page being read, much less a whole book.

His sleep was frequently interrupted. He would awaken, crying uncontrollably, jolted awake by some unseen horror. Hours would pass before he was calm enough to drift back to sleep, if he were able to go back to sleep at all.

His diet was very limited. He ate black or kidney beans, cooked or raw carrots, apples or grapes, raisins, fast food french fries, and homemade casein-free bread that I baked for him. If the food wasn't immediately recognizable, it remained untouched. I marveled at the seemingly purposeful selection of only healthy foods, except for his favorite food, french fries. Why does he crave them, I wondered, when all the other foods he chooses to eat are such healthy foods?

He would not play with any toys. If we handed a stuffed animal to him, he would throw it without even looking at it. He would allow me to hug him, but he held his body stiff and rigid, with his arms at his sides. By this time, he would not make eye contact, except when being rocked to sleep at night. He still had eyes that looked right into your soul.

Benjamin reached the point where he was extremely sensitive to all medications. If I had to give him a course of antibiotics, he would throw tantrums and act out for up to two weeks after the last dosage. When he became ill with croup and was having some difficulty breathing, his pediatrician was not available, but his colleague wanted to prescribe oral steroids. I expressed great concern at giving steroids to a child who was so sensitive.

The pediatrician retorted, "You can give it to him now, or if you don't, we can give it to him intravenously tomorrow when we have to admit him to the hospital."

I let fear get the best of me, and took the prescription. There is a well-known side effect of steroids, called roid rage. After this experience, I could understand why professional athletes take steroids. Nothing could stand in the way of what Benjamin wanted. He was extremely aggressive, trying to knock me down, throwing things, and acting extremely angry. My sweet and gentle boy turned into a raging maniac. The effect lasted for ten days. The effect is supposed to occur only if steroids are taken for ten days or more. Benjamin received only two days of medication. I wanted so badly to leave him on the pediatrician's doorstep for a few days!

At that time Benjamin's daily routine was very predictable. He would wake up in the morning and go straight to the playroom to turn on the television and VCR. He would watch several of his favorite videos while jumping on his small trampoline. I would drag him away from the television to dress him. He would sit limply on his dresser as I pulled off his pajamas and dressed him in clean clothes. He would wince as I brushed his hair and teeth. My mother and stepfather would pick him up and take him to the local mall to walk; there he would eat an entire order of fast-food french fries. When he returned home, he would watch videos and jump on the trampoline until lunchtime. He would eat his standard fare of beans, fruits, and vegetables, then return to watching his videos, or run endlessly in our backyard until I came and got him. This continued until something forced its way into his awareness, such as the need for a diaper change.

Then, after dinner, the dressing routine, this time into his pajamas, would repeat itself.

The only time he acknowledged me was when he needed something; then he would cry or fuss or pull at me to try and indicate what he wanted. Caring for Benjamin was more like caring for a small puppy. When he cried, I tried everything to figure out what he wanted. My world was full of hunches and guesses as to what he wanted or needed at any given moment. I ran in circles, trying to make him more comfortable and keep him happy. There were days that I didn't eat a bite of food until my husband returned home from work. The minute I would try to do anything else, the crying and fussing would start, and I would begin the frantic guessing game. If I didn't do my job well, then he would lie down, kicking and screaming, until I figured out what he needed. It took me quite some time just to figure out that when he demonstrated these behaviors, he was trying to tell me that he needed something.

I was caring for an infant in the body of a two-year-old. Sometimes I felt more like a servant chained to a prisoner than a mother staying home with a child. I knew that I was physically and emotionally exhausted when my daughter approached me one day with her soft, pink, lovey doll named Rosie. Rosie was her constant companion and an absolute necessity for sleeping at night.

Handing the doll to me, Karis looked into my eyes saying, "Here, Mommy. You keep Rosie. You need her more than I do."

I remembered reading somewhere that when a child is asked to define "God," the child is most likely to equate god with their favorite lovey item. In her characteristically kind and selfless manner, Karis was willing to give up her "God" in order to comfort me.

When I left Benjamin with my husband or my mother, he often sobbed inconsolably. The time we spent together was his security blanket, even though many times I couldn't even figure out what he wanted. We were both imprisoned by his world. He couldn't get out, and I couldn't find a way in.

When Benjamin was about two and a half years old, I attempted to enroll him in a mother's day out program in a local church. I left him there the first day, not expecting any problems. After all, my daughter had gone part-time to a preschool and adapted just fine. Upon arriving to pick up Benjamin at the church, the teacher took me aside and said that they didn't think that Benjamin was ready for the two- to three-year-old class, and they suggested that he be enrolled in the younger class for 18-month-old children. He was unable to follow directions and participate in the activities and his inability to switch from one activity to the next was disruptive to the class. I removed him from the program, rationalizing that his behavior was due to the fact that he had never been placed in any type of preschool situation before. After all, I thought, those other children had probably been in daycare since birth. Denial can be such a powerful thing.

2 The Allergies

Each journey begins with a single step.

—Adam

At ten weeks old we first saw that something was awry in our little boy. He broke out in hives after I supplemented with baby formula. He had huge raised, angry-looking welts all over his tiny body, and he screamed. He really screamed. The pediatrician said that he was probably allergic to milk, so I began supplementing with soy formula. That seemed to do the trick. At Benjamin's next appointment, I mentioned my amazement that he could be so allergic to cow's milk. The pediatrician said that a milk tolerance test was necessary to document Benjamin's file. I expressed my concern with deliberately giving him milk.

Once Benjamin found the wooden stick from an ice-cream treat that had been licked clean by his sister. Within seconds of touching the stick to his face, huge red, raised welts appeared on his face. I reminded the doctor of the time we brought Benjamin in after he ate a small piece of a cheese puff that he had found on the floor. He was not as concerned as my husband and I were though, because by the time the doctor arrived, over an hour after the offending cheese puff had been consumed, Benjamin's reaction had somewhat subsided.

The doctor countered by telling me that a blood test failed to reveal a severe milk allergy. Against my better judgment, I made the appointment, bringing a small bottle of milk purchased at the nearby convenience store. After all, in my mind, the doctor was the ultimate authority on my child's health. Benjamin began projectile vomiting after the first few swallows of milk. After the cheese puff incident, I was only mildly surprised at this reaction, but became alarmed when I saw the doctor's response and two shots of adrenaline were necessary to stop the reaction.

As my apologetic pediatrician later related to me, I brought a healthy child into the office that day and left with a very sick child. When I asked him what could be done about the allergy, he told me that Benjamin's reaction was among the worst he had seen in more than 25 years of practice. I was instructed to keep everything containing the milk protein casein away from Benjamin. He suggested that I wait several years and have Benjamin take allergy shots, so that he would not go into anaphylactic shock in the school cafeteria when he started school. He said that there was virtually no hope of him ever outgrowing an allergy that was this severe.

Benjamin had a patch of eczema on his cheek almost from the time he was born. We now believe that this was a slight allergic reaction to breast milk and even the soy formula he was given his first year.

Benjamin suffered from airborne allergies, too. He constantly had a runny nose. On one occasion, my husband rented a car, and my daughter wanted to ride in it. When we got into it, I noticed a rather strong smell of upholstery protectant. Benjamin was ill for three days. He became ill from running in a friend's yard where fresh cedar chips had been placed. On another occasion, he became ill when visiting San Antonio when cedar and ash levels were particularly high and remained sick for days. I dusted a large, very high shelf in our home and he was ill for a week. He slept with a vaporizer in his room every night for the first several years of his life.

I began baking bread for Benjamin. After experiencing his severe reaction to milk, I was afraid that the machinery used in commercial bakeries could contaminate even products that didn't contain casein. He ate nothing but food prepared at home. An infrequent trip to a restaurant involved packing all of his food into his diaper bag. Trips to areas where other children played were exhausting. I had to be aware of all of the other children's food and drinks. I became aware of how common it was for mothers to bring milk for their children in those little child sippy cups. Benjamin could snatch and drink from another child's cup before I could move two feet in his direction to retrieve it. I began having to follow directly behind him while he was playing if food was present. When he wasn't stealing drinks, he was engaging in his second most favorite activity, stealing french fries from the plates of the people sitting in the common eating area of our local mall.

3 The Diagnosis

Love's direction guards us not against grief but against a dark-
ening of the heart.

—John Donne

By the time Benjamin was two and a half, we were very concerned
by his lack of speech. He had said a few words early on, but was not progressing at anywhere near the rate our daughter had. Filling out the
forms in the pediatrician's office detailing the usual childhood milestones, I began to realize that Benjamin was lagging very far behind in
his speech and social interaction. The milestones of concern were an
increase in the number of words spoken and included the combining
of several words. Benjamin had not said a word in almost a year.

His grandmother picked him up after one of those rare occasions
when she left him at a drop-in childcare center for a few hours.
Benjamin would tolerate staying at the center for a short time, provided that his sister and his beloved french fries were present. A student
worker asked my mother if he was autistic. We were dumbfounded that
someone would ask such a question. Of course our beautiful boy was
not autistic.

As the pediatrician indicated in response to my concerns, he was
just a boy, and boys normally do not progress as quickly as girls. He

also pointed out that my very verbal daughter probably did the talking for him, so he just did not have a need to talk. To be on the safe side, I decided to contact a state agency that dealt with child development concerns. I figured that I could at least start him in speech therapy, even though his pediatrician was not concerned. In the meantime, a friend, who is an ear, nose, and throat surgeon, suggested that we bring Benjamin in to check his ears and his hearing. He did not pass the preliminary test, which requires a child to react physically to certain sounds. He had some fluid in his ears, so we decided to have tubes put in his ears. While he was under the anesthesia, the doctor performed an auditory brain stem response test. The test revealed that his brain was reacting within the normal range to sound, even if his body wasn't. Benjamin's hearing wasn't the problem.

A few weeks later, the state agency sent a speech therapist to our home to do an evaluation. Benjamin refused to look at her or stay in one place long enough for her to do an assessment. I finally placed him in his high chair, fastening a strap around his waist to keep him secure. He turned his body completely away from the therapist. The high chair was the kind that has plastic side panels that snap forward and backward. He turned sideways and clicked the panels back and forth repeatedly. I had not realized until that day that he exhibited avoidance behavior. She concluded that he displayed some "autistic-like symptoms" and that we should take him back to our pediatrician for a diagnosis.

A physical beating would have felt better than the shock that reverberated throughout my body upon hearing those words. At a friend's suggestion, we changed to a different pediatrician and made an appointment with an educational neuropsychologist to get more information about autism spectrum disorders.

Within a few days we met with the neuropsychologist, who had asked to meet with us without Benjamin. She asked us about Benjamin's symptoms, then began talking about how behavior disorders are typically handled by the use of medications. I was aware that there was little research on the safety of brain-altering drugs used on children. When I was a juvenile prosecutor, I had often wondered about the long-term consequences of exposing a developing brain to powerful psychiatric medications. When I expressed concern about giving medications to a child, especially one with extreme sensitivities, she replied that he had to be able to "sit still and learn" and indicated that in her experience there were no other options.

Visions of the children diagnosed with attention-deficit/hyperactivity disorder that I had worked with when I was a juvenile prosecutor flashed before my eyes—the nice, compliant children on Ritalin and various other drugs, with their sleepy, vacant eyes and blank affect. The only people that seemed happy were the teachers who could now control them, and the parents who reported that their lives were now much easier. The children just seemed to want to die. Many tried their best to do just that.

My husband and I left the meeting outraged and fearful. I just couldn't understand the reasoning in drugging Benjamin for everyone else's convenience when no one could even tell us why he was the way he was. I vowed that day that if I had to make a choice between medicating Benjamin and taking care of him for the rest of my life, then I would do the latter. I didn't care what anyone else thought had to be done. Slowly, I started to develop a plan of action. First, I knew that I must find ways to make him more comfortable in his body that didn't include dulling his senses with medications. Then, I would try to figure out what capabilities Benjamin actually possessed. Understanding Benjamin would become my passion. He would become the most important case of my life.

We waited impatiently for the few days to elapse before our appointment with the new pediatrician. He observed Benjamin, asked numerous questions, then told us that a diagnosis of an autism spectrum disorder is achieved not by finding a particular gene or problem with a child's blood or body. It is instead achieved when a child exhibits a group of characteristics or behaviors and a blood test rules out two known genetic abnormalities with similar symptoms: fragile X syndrome and Klinefelter's syndrome. If these two disorders were ruled out by a blood test, then Benjamin's default diagnosis would likely be pervasive developmental disorder not otherwise specified (PDD-NOS), which is a disorder within the range of autism spectrum disorders. Autism spectrum disorders are characterized by a group of symptoms rather than a pinpointed cause. My husband took Benjamin to our local hospital for the necessary blood test. It would take weeks to get the results.

Upon arriving home, I immediately began researching autism spectrum disorders, fragile X syndrome, and Klinefelter's syndrome. My husband's brother-in-law, who is a psychiatrist, assured us that Benjamin probably didn't have Klinefelter's syndrome because he did not exhibit the physical characteristics of the disease. After researching the syndrome, I also felt certain that the test would not reveal this syndrome. When I began to research fragile X and Klinefelter's syndromes, my heart sank as I read that boys who suffer from Klinefelter's syndrome are typically sterile.

I found that autism is described as a "lifelong brain disorder with very severe problems communicating, responding to surroundings, and forming relationships."[1] The incidence of autism is "exploding." It is now estimated that as many as 1 in 250 children suffer from some form of the disorder.[2] Most will require lifelong care and cannot live independently. More than half of autistic children will never speak. Many of them will never be able to look at their parents and tell them that they love them.

Autistic children have been described as being self-absorbed, lost in a fantasy world, or attempting to escape reality. Possessing no sense of others, autistic children are thought to feel virtually alone in the world.

I found that although many experts believe that autism is a biological disorder, caused by organic rather than psychological causes, the American Psychiatric Association's criteria remain the standard for an autism diagnosis, and it is still considered a mental disorder.

According to the *Diagnostic and Statistical Manual of Mental Disorders-Fourth Edition* (DSM-IV), for a diagnosis of autism, a person must exhibit at least six characteristics from the three areas delineated below, with at least two from the first category and one each from the other two categories.[3]

• Impairment in social interaction
  impairment in nonverbal behaviors related to social interaction, such as eye contact and facial expression
  failure to develop peer relationships
  lack of spontaneous sharing of enjoyment or interests, as evidenced by showing or pointing out objects
  lack of social or emotional reciprocity

- Impairment in communication
  delayed or nonexistent language development
  impairment in conversation abilities if language is present
  stereotypic, repetitive language or idiosyncratic language
  lack of make-believe or social imitative play

- Repetitive and stereotyped behavior, interests, and activities
  abnormally intense preoccupation with one or more interests
  seemingly inflexible adherence to routines or rituals
  stereotyped and repetitive mannerisms, such as hand or finger
    flapping or twisting, or whole-body movements
  preoccupation with object parts

Although Benjamin seemed to exhibit more than six characteristics outlined in the manual, his pediatrician had indicated that pervasive developmental disorder would probably be his diagnosis. From the same manual under the category pervasive developmental disorders, I discovered that this diagnosis is achieved when a child falls short of exhibiting characteristics in all three categories. The manual listed the following general characteristics of autism spectrum disorders, which I found to be quite disturbing:

- Range of behavior symptoms, including hyperactivity, short attention span, impulsivity, aggressiveness, self-injurious behaviors, and in young children, temper tantrums.

- In most cases, there is an associated diagnosis of Mental Retardation, commonly in the moderate range (IQ 35–50). Approximately 75 percent of children with Autistic Disorder function at a retarded level.

- [O]nly a small percentage of individuals with the disorder go on as adults to live and work independently.[4]

The outcome for individuals diagnosed with this disorder is considered to be poor in 61 to 73 percent of cases, with 39 to 54 percent of the children being institutionalized. The outcome is good in 5 to 15 percent of cases.

Benjamin's caseworker gave me the article "The Early Origins of Autism" by Patricia M. Rodier. The article outlined in more simple language three diagnostic categories for a diagnosis of an autism spectrum disorder:*

Impairment of Social Interaction: Failure to use eye contact, facial expression, or gestures to regulate social interaction; failure to seek comfort; failure to develop relationships with peers.

Impairment of Communication: Failure to use spoken language, without compensating by gesture; deficit in initiating or sustaining a conversation, despite adequate speech; aberrant language (for example, repeating a question instead of replying).

Restricted and Repetitive Interests and Behaviors: Abnormally intense preoccupation with one subject or activity; distress over change; insistence on routines or rituals with no purpose; repetitive movements, such as hand flapping.

A diagnosis of autism requires that the patient exhibit abnormal behaviors in the above three categories and have especially notable deficits in the category of social interaction. In addition, clinicians have identified several related disorders that share some of the behavioral features of autism but have different emphases or additional symptoms. For example, pervasive developmental disorder not otherwise specified (PDD-NOS) denotes patients who miss fulfilling the autism criteria in one of the three categories.[5]

I realized much later that Benjamin, in fact, did meet criteria in all three categories. Medical professionals are hesitant to label very young children as autistic, however, and prefer to use the PDD-NOS label, which is much more ambiguous and acceptable to most parents. I was beginning to realize that despite many different theories about the causes of autism spectrum disorders, no one really knew

---

*From "The Early Origins of Autism" by Patricia M. Rodier. Copyright © 2000 by Scientific American, Inc. All rights reserved.

what this disorder was or why these children exhibited these behaviors. The autism spectrum disorder bin is the one that a child is dumped into when nothing else fits.

Rodier's article continued by outlining several physical anomalies that accompany the disorder, including differences that have been noted in the brain stem of persons diagnosed with the disorder and similarities in physical facial characteristics. These children tend to have corners of the mouth that are low compared with the center of the upper lip, the tops of the ears flop over, and the ears are a bit lower than normal and have an almost square shape. The article also noted that people with autism have often been described as unusually attractive. As the photocopy of the article was dark and the pictures were unclear, I rushed to our computer to look the article up online. I found the page showing the face of the autistic child.

I glanced beside the computer at the close-up head and shoulders photo of Benjamin and Karis that we had sent as a Christmas card to all our friends and family. It was taken when Karis was two and a half, and Benjamin was just three months old. I was so proud of the photo. Karis was striking with her huge brown eyes and straight auburn hair. Benjamin's piercing blue eyes highlighted his angelic face. Then I looked at his ears. Oh my God, I thought. It's really true. How could I have been so stupid? The tops of Benjamin's ears flopped over slightly, just as the boy's in the article did. He looks like a poster boy for autism, I thought. I felt the familiar jolt in my stomach and the fear creeping back into my chest, my eyes once again filling with tears. I forced myself to take another look. He's still incredibly beautiful, I thought, and his eyes spoke volumes even as a baby, I recalled. Keep looking for the positive, I told myself, as I wiped away the tears with the back of my hand and continued scanning the article.

When the test results arrived three weeks later, they ruled out both fragile X and Klinefelter's syndromes. By default, Benjamin was dumped into the bin of pervasive developmental disorder not otherwise specified.

I found out much later about a checklist of key social, emotional, and communication milestones developed by First Signs, an organization located in Merrimac, Massachusetts, that is dedicated to educating parents and physicians about the early warning signs of autism and other developmental disorders. This checklist allows parents and physicians to work together to chart a child's developmental progress. The following milestones should be used as discussion points between a parent and a child's physician at the child's well visit to determine if an 18-month-old child is progressing normally:

Does Your Baby . . . At 18 Months:

• Use lots of gestures with words to get needs met, like pointing or taking you by the hand and saying, "want juice"?

• Use at least four different consonants in babbling or words, such as m, n, p, b, t, and d?

• Use and understand at least ten words?

• Show that he or she knows the names of familiar people or body parts by pointing to or looking at them when they are named?

• Do simple pretend play, like feeding a doll or stuffed animal, and attracting your attention by looking up at you?[6]

At two and a half, Benjamin was unable to perform any of these actions.

After we met with the pediatrician and Benjamin had his blood drawn, I became numb with grief, unwilling to fully comprehend the finality of Benjamin's life sentence of autism. I cried for a day and half, sitting numbly on our family room couch, mired in the hollow emptiness of fear and dread. My daughter, sensing my despair, once again brought me her favorite doll, Rosie, and I clutched onto it as if it were a life raft from God.

My husband remained completely calm, caring for the children and handling the household. On the second day, he said to me in his characteristically optimistic manner, "I know that Benjamin will be okay. Just let me know when you're finished."

I just couldn't shake the overwhelming feeling of terror. I knew that everything I thought for certain about my world was going to change. I knew that my life as I had been living it was over. I was terrified of confronting this change, but knew that there was nothing that I could do to stop its relentless advance. My head reeled and my heart ached. There was no escape, no secret trapdoor through which I could quietly slip. For the first time in my life, I was in a situation that I could not control. I knew that there was no way I could think my way out of this one. I felt helplessly and hopelessly stuck.

On the evening of the second day, I began to feel the following words and concepts forming in my mind, as if I were perceiving them from someplace outside myself:

Guided in our every step
Breathing in each labored breath
I struggled with the burden of knowing
Labels given to his world of silence
But the beautiful face I gaze upon
Could never be seen as withdrawn
To a mother who sees the depth within
In eyes that gaze upon the wind
I know our lives will always differ
From this day forward without a whimper
To see the spirit that's always been free
One puts away his misery
And follows this where destiny flows
Down any path my beautiful boy goes.

I was puzzled by the words rushing into my head. I had never written a poem in all my life, choosing instead to write technical, factual papers on the law. The words came to me quickly and in their final form. In less than a minute, I typed the words into our computer. Then I went to bed and, for the first time since I heard the word "autism," slipped into a deep, restful sleep.

When I awoke the next morning, my head was clear and the fog had lifted. I began to realize that what I had been struggling with was not whether Benjamin would be okay, but with the idea of having a less than perfect child. I was afraid of having a child who took the "short bus" to school. My husband could not understand my reaction because he had already accepted him the way he was. I had not. I was not really concerned about the quality of Benjamin's life. He could find pure bliss in the breaking of the waves, or the passing of the morning school bus.

I realized that by holding on to the idea that my children were supposed to fit society's definition of normal, rather than accepting *what is*,[7] I was setting myself up for depression, repression, and pain. I knew I would have to completely and unequivocally accept Benjamin's condition, whatever it ultimately was, in order to avoid the pain.

Up until this point in my life, I had come to the conclusion that everything in my life, both good and bad, had happened to me for a reason. Could I still hold this belief when it involved my child? Did I really believe this, or was this something to be believed when it was someone else facing a time of pain and crisis, something you think when someone else encounters difficulty? It makes so much sense when it isn't you staring into the face of a major life crisis. I made the decision to surrender this situation to a higher power. I did not know if Benjamin was mentally retarded or if he would ever be able to live independently as an adult. It didn't matter. Aside from his apparent bodily discomfort, he wasn't in any real pain. He was my son. I knew I could love and accept him whether he ever improved or not.

Still I knew that most of the time, life must be incredibly frustrating for him. My instincts told me that there was so much waiting inside that head, that beautiful, blond, curly head with the penetrating blue eyes, those eyes that were always speaking to me, pleading with me. I was terrified that Benjamin might think that this had all been a huge mistake.

While working as a juvenile prosecutor, occasionally I would work with children who were involved with social services, due to their unfortunate family situations. These children were often labeled "failure to thrive." There were no detectable physical problems with these children, but it seemed that many times they were just silently slipping away. Their situations were just too much for their small bodies to bear. With the instinct of a damaged cell, they would slip into aptosis, silently turning on the suicide program. I feared that Benjamin, too, would find all of this too much to bear, and slowly begin slipping away from me and away from this whole frustrating situation. I feared that like an underqualified, unprepared, and disgruntled employee trying to make a go of it at a difficult new job, he would locate his time card, slide it in until it clicked, proving that he showed up for the last, frustrating, incomprehensible day, and quietly slip out the door, never to be seen or heard from again.

"Just stay with me buddy," I'd think to myself. "I promise you I'll figure it out. Just stay with me." I couldn't even bear to think about life without him.

Soon after Benjamin's diagnosis, I wrote a short story for Karis to help her deal with the frustration of living with an autistic brother. I titled it, "Where Oh Where Is Brother Ben?" I didn't realize it at the time, but it was very descriptive of Benjamin's daily existence on many levels. We never knew where we would find Benjamin, either his physical body or the focus of his awareness. Sometimes it just seemed as if no one was at home.

I could certainly relate to the words of a father of a ten-year-old autistic boy: "Our son looks so perfectly normal. It's like looking at a piece of jewelry under glass. He's a bright, beautiful child, but we just can't break through."[8]

When thinking about an autistic child, the phrases that first come to mind are that the child is "somewhere else," living "out there," or "locked in his own world." Attempts are made to "bring the child back into our world." Some parents describe their children being dragged, kicking and screaming, into a life in the world.

My journey would not involve dragging Benjamin into my world. I had no desire to do that. I would not engage in a battle with his condition. I felt that to engage in a battle, I had to at least know what it was that I was fighting. All I knew was that he had a diagnosis of a condition that no one seemed to know very much about.

Instinctively, I felt that that there was much more to this situation than what I was consciously aware of. I knew my only battle was to be one of understanding. I knew that if an answer existed in the medical or scientific realm, I could find it and understand it. The problem was that my research revealed that there was nothing that the medical community could offer me that would begin to explain it. All the conventional medicine in the world couldn't help me. I instinctively knew that I had to learn enough about Benjamin's world to see if he could be coaxed into mine. The only way I knew how to do this was to begin to trust my intuition and ask to be shown the nature of his condition. I knew that I would have to go beyond conventional science and reason to a place where I could "see" and "understand" what was not immediately apparent. I knew that I must go back in time, to that place I had trusted almost 20 years ago.

4 The Challenges and Differences

I know people by their "edges." Edges have nothing to do with
interpretation or surface actions or words. Edges are the "being-
ness" beyond the surface "appearance," the truth beyond the
facade. They are the foundations of selfhood; its body without
the clothes or overlay that either fit it or disguise it. Edges told
me who my own edges were compatible with; a kind of soul dia-
logue that is based on feel, not on thought. I was surrounded by
an external world of constructed egos and minds and bodies, of
lives and trends. But all I saw were souls and everything else was
transient background information which I got trained to take
account of long after other people had already acquired the
mental capacity to take account of it instantly, as their fore-
ground.
—*Donna Williams,* Autism and Sensing: The Unlost Instinct, *1999*

Sometimes I think what a cruel joke it is. I can imagine in the great
cosmic scheme of things a plan being formed, a plan where the child
coming into the world will be so different, so unique that the child
will not respond to conventional treatments or traditional schooling.
The child will be hypersensitive to smells, sounds, tastes, colors, electromagnetic and magnetic fields. Things that are proven beneficial to

other children will have devastating effects on this child. The child will have no fears of his own. The child will know your thoughts and what is in your heart. He'll react to your emotions and take your fears, turning them up a notch. The child will straddle many worlds at once.

One night in my dreams, the universe spoke directly to me.

"The only way to get through to this child is to work on yourself," the universe said. "You'll have to surrender many beliefs. You'll have to suspend many judgments. You'll have to see, really see what is before you. You must work on yourself or you will not understand. Some will think that the child is broken and needs to be fixed. His challenges will come from what he encounters here, not the attributes he came here with. You must undo the damage, then unconditionally accept what remains."

My awareness zoomed to a woman standing in a long hallway, dressed only in pajamas, blanket wrapped around her shoulders, tears streaming down her face. I stood in line to put myself in one of the most stressful positions possible, she was thinking, and now you are telling me it's time to work on myself? Yeah, she thought, I really feel like doing that. Especially when the thoughts of the day are train 'em, drug 'em, or put 'em away. Even this is more acceptable than what you are telling me to do.

"It's your choice. You can continue on as if there is no hope, but he is in your hands," the universe continued.

The woman was reminded of a quote by Sir Winston Churchill: "Most people, sometime in their lives, stumble across truth. And most jump up, brush themselves off, and hurry on about their business as if nothing had happened."

The realization began to sink in of the times she had done this in the past. Suddenly, the woman and I merged into one, and I realized that I was watching myself as the woman in the dream.

"I'll guide you and help you," the universe added.

"But you can't get up with him and rock him for hours when the sleep won't come," I replied.

"I'll send you two helpers, your husband and your daughter," the universe assured me.

An image of a tall, athletic, blond Norwegian appeared. He was tossing a small boy, a mirror image of himself. Up into the air went the boy, giggling and screaming with such glee that it seemed that catching his breath would be impossible. This doesn't look so difficult or scary, I thought.

Another image appeared, of a tall, dark-haired girl, about six years old, with my large brown eyes. She was wise beyond her years. She was talking to the boy, her attention transfixed on his every move.

"Good job, Benji," she exclaimed. "Momma, momma, he said *a*, he said *a*. I can't believe it, he knows what an *a* is," she said. "Gimme a hug, Benji, you did so well," she exclaimed. "Good job, Benji."

Maybe I can do this, I thought, then the familiar fear crept in. "What about my doubts and fears?" I asked.

"I'll send others to you, who can reassure you and guide you. They'll be similar to your son but much older and so remarkable that they will make the choice much easier for you to make," the universe answered.

"They'd better be DAMN GOOD," I replied.

What was the truth about Benjamin? Truth is that which empowers you, but cannot do harm. I had to find this truth.

Before Benjamin was diagnosed, he would go on outings with my mother and stepfather to our local mall to walk, before the stores opened. They would walk a few rounds down the corridors of the mall, pushing Benjamin in a stroller, then stop in the food court for french fries and to let Benjamin play in the children's play area. They would have to follow the same routine each time or Benjamin would get very upset. They could not go to the play area first before walking or he would cry and start pushing the stroller to indicate that he wanted to walk. If there were no french fries ready at the fast-food counter, he would scream. If they started walking from a different starting point, a tantrum would follow. They had a difficult time keeping him inside the play area. He liked to run outside the play area and find doors to open and shut. If you tried to move him, a full-blown screaming scene followed. Whatever Benjamin was focused on, he wanted to be left alone to focus on it, or an ordeal was sure to follow. Talking to him was like talking to a brick. There was no sign that he had any understanding of anything that was said. When a tantrum ensued, the only recourse was to put him in his stroller and leave with him, his screams reverberating off the walls of the long corridors. The choice was to let him do whatever he was focused upon or deal with a tantrum.

The difficult part of this stage in his life was that we had no idea what he understood, if anything, about the situation we were exposing him to. Nothing mattered except the thing he was focused on. It was his entire world at that moment. The situation would get even more difficult when I would try to take him to the same mall to shop. He expected sameness and routine. He couldn't grasp that this was a different situation where we would do different activities. He had a tape in his head of how things were to transpire, and you couldn't alter the tape. I think that at this time he couldn't grasp change because virtually no one else existed in his reality, including me. Unless he was focused on my face, he wasn't aware that I existed. His reality was the focus of his awareness at that particular time. He had virtually no awareness of anyone else, except to the extent that they somehow played a part in his tape. He practically ignored his sister, except if she inserted herself into his tape. A fun activity that she was engaging in while trying to include him might temporarily bring her into his awareness, but it was fleeting and rare.

His lack of awareness was beyond frustrating. An alien, who at first blush appeared quite human, had been unleashed in our family, and no one had any useful suggestions on how to deal with him. As he was so large and strong, he was particularly difficult to manage. We began to control carefully each situation that Benjamin was exposed to in order to minimize the behaviors with which we had to deal. One parent would do things with our daughter, and the other would be assigned to monitor Benjamin's world. We never planned outings for the four of us because they would always result in disaster. Benjamin's behavior made any activity virtually impossible. We became prisoners in Benjamin's world, mindlessly following the same patterns, day after day, because he couldn't tolerate any change.

During this time, he demonstrated a great deal of sensitivity in his body. He hated to have his teeth brushed. The only way he would open his mouth was if I sang to him while I tried to brush his teeth. I still sing musical scales while brushing his teeth. He appeared to get lost in the music, instead of focusing on the sensation of being brushed. When he was very young, he refused to allow me to clip his fingernails and toenails. I would have to steal into his room at night and clip his fingernails and toenails while he was sleeping.

Often he would seem to be in a state of pure bliss. He would run to his bed, lie down with his face buried in his pillow with his arms straight down by his side. He would gently bounce his body on the bed. We called this his "dolphin kick" because the movement seemed to mimic the movement of a dolphin in the water. Sometimes he would be laughing or verbalizing sounds but it was apparent that his dolphin kick was the equivalent of other children's jumping up and down for joy.

He had an extremely limited diet. He would eat only certain fruits, carrots, and two kinds of beans, black beans or kidney beans. Once we were able to get his milk allergy under control, he started eating Cheerios. Later I was amazed to discover that Benjamin's self-selected diet was almost a perfect macrobiotic diet. A macrobiotic diet is often encouraged for people with compromised immune systems. Many physicians recommend the diet when someone is diagnosed with cancer or an autoimmune disease. Benjamin had self-selected a diet that was the least taxing on his body. One facet of the macrobiotic diet is the elimination of meat from the diet. Benjamin has always refused to eat any kind of meat, in any form.

I often found that Benjamin was mirroring my moods. If I woke up particularly out of sorts, Benjamin would be out of sorts, too. If I were particularly happy, he would be happy, too. When I got irritated, he became very irritated. The more irritated I became, the more irritated Benjamin became. We all had to become very clear about what we were feeling, and why. Any fears that we experienced were immediately picked up and volleyed back to us like atomic tennis balls. Any unspoken hostilities materialized in the behavior of our little boy. We were forced to look at our fears, name them, pick them apart, and destroy them. The process was painstaking, excruciating, and thorough.

Looking at our feelings was the only way to eliminate them, thus allowing some semblance of a normal life. I would work through my feelings of frustration and fear, then my husband would return from his business travels, and the process would begin all over again. Benjamin proceeded with the skill of a surgeon, locating, dissecting, and destroying each part of us that stood in the way of our understanding. We were constantly asking each other, "What are you feeling?" "Why are you frustrated?" "Why do you care what others think about Benjamin's condition?" "What is really going on here?" There was no room for dishonesty. The soothsayer stood before us. If there was anger, it had to be rooted out or it would be acted upon. If there was frustration, it had to be identified. Slowly, we began to realize that in working on each of our own personal issues, we were throwing fewer and fewer grenades into the environment for Benjamin to deal with. He was somehow reading our emotions and sometimes even our thoughts before there were any outward signs.

Sometimes I felt that I had more in common with Superman's fictitious parents than with parents of normal children. I was always aware, searching and ferreting out the hidden Kryptonite that might paralyze my son. I was always analyzing, then working this massive jigsaw puzzle called autism, trying to fit the pieces together so that I could see the whole picture with clarity.

Any doubts we had about whether Benjamin was mirroring the emotional state of others were resolved one day when we boarded the light rail train near our home in Silicon Valley for a short trip. As the doors opened, Benjamin rushed to the only open seat next to the window, directly behind a homeless woman. I noticed her becoming uncomfortable as Benjamin kneeled beside the window. She fidgeted in her chair. Benjamin began to shout loudly one-syllable sounds, similar to a person with Tourette's syndrome. He never does this unless he is very uncomfortable, and he had never demonstrated this type of behavior on the train. Ordinarily, the train has a very calming effect on him as he gazes out the window and watches the doors open and close at each stop. As people boarded the train, the woman blocked the empty seat next to her with her arm, obviously fearing close contact from anyone sitting next to her. Benjamin became more and more agitated. She turned and glared briefly at Benjamin. Suddenly, with his desperation rising, he screamed, "red devil, red devil, red devil." My husband looked at me with a startled expression. There was no doubt in either of our minds that Benjamin had picked up on the woman's tortured state of mind. Finally, we reached our station and the woman continued on her way. Benjamin's behavior began to return to normal.

We began to realize that Benjamin was consistently acting on the things that others were feeling but not expressing. My husband and I approached an upscale restaurant with outdoor seating. As we stood in the doorway with Benjamin in tow, the waitstaff ignored us. I seethed inside as we continued to be ignored. Benjamin will never wait this long, I thought to myself, my discomfort increasing.

"Aaaarrrrrgh," Benjamin screamed directly into the open door of the restaurant.

"May I help you," a startled employee blurted out as he made a rush toward us.

"Could we please be seated outside," I asked, sensing that the chances for success would be greater there.

"Certainly," the waitperson replied.

Boy, that is certainly what I wanted to do, Benjamin, I thought. I made a mental note not to allow myself to get so irritated in the future.

A sympathetic waiter who was the father of a small child appeared. Benjamin was relaxed and comfortable. The man continued to address Benjamin, even when he didn't respond, and we had a relatively normal dinner—that is, until Benjamin succeeded in falling backward in his chair, landing with a thud on the concrete. We scooped him up and carried him sobbing to the train. "At least we got to eat this time," my husband mused.

Benjamin displayed some self-stimulatory behavior. Stereotyptic or self-stimulatory behavior refers to repetitive body movements or the repetitive movement of objects. This behavior, often referred to as "stimming" is common in many individuals with developmental disabilities; however, it appears to be more common in autism. In fact, if a person with another developmental disability exhibits a form of self-stimulatory behavior, often the person is also labeled as having autistic characteristics. Benjamin would spontaneously look at certain things with a very excited look on his face, while making some repetitive hand movements. He had a tendency to thrust his arms backward and engage in hand flapping while thrusting his torso slightly forward. Occasionally, he would smell objects or people. He engaged in hand flapping when he was watching water swirl down the drain, when he was watching the wheels of the train as it accelerated, when noticing a particular area of a person's body, or when looking at certain works of art.

In "Stereotypic (Self-Stimulatory) Behavior" by Stephen M. Edelson, Ph.D., stereotypy is described as a disorder involving any one or all five senses as follows:[1]

Sense	Stereotypic Behaviors
Visual	staring at lights, repetitive blinking, moving fingers in front of the eyes, hand flapping
Auditory	tapping ears, snapping fingers, making vocal sounds
Tactile	rubbing the skin with one's hands or with another object, scratching
Vestibular	rocking front to back, rocking side-to-side
Taste	placing body parts or objects in one's mouth, licking objects
Smell	smelling objects, sniffing people

Researchers have suggested various reasons why a person may engage in stereotypic behaviors. One set of theories suggests that a person is hyposensitive and, thus, such behaviors provide the person with sensory stimulation. According to this theory, some dysfunctional system in the brain or periphery causes the body to crave stimulation, and the person engages in these behaviors to excite or arouse the nervous system. One specific theory states that these behaviors release beta-endorphins, which are endogenous opiate-like substances in the body, and provide the person with some form of internal pleasure.

Another set of theories states that a person is hypersensitive, and these behaviors are exhibited to calm a person. The environment is too stimulating and the person is in a state of sensory overload. As a result, the individual engages in these behaviors to block out the overstimulating environment; and his/her attention becomes focused inwardly.

Researchers have shown that stereotypic behaviors interfere with attention and learning, but have found that these behaviors serve as effective positive reinforcement if a person is allowed to engage in these behaviors after completing a task. Various methods are used to reduce or eliminate stereotypic behaviors, such as exercise or providing an individual with a more socially appropriate alternative behavior. Drugs may also be used to reduce these behaviors; however, it is not clear whether the drugs actually reduce the behaviors directly by providing internal arousal or indirectly by slowing down one's overall motor movement.[2]

I was confused by these explanations of why "stimming" occurs in autistic children. In Benjamin's case, he only "stimmed" when looking at certain things, usually something that created lots of whirling energy. Water swirling down the drain, large trucks passing on the street, the spinning of train wheels on the track resulted in "stimming." He wasn't creating these situations in order to "stim," he just "stimmed" when he perceived them. If he was "stimming" because of sensory overload, why would these particular situations cause overload to his system, when they didn't cause it in mine, or anyone else's who isn't autistic? He seemed to be seeing or sensing something of which I wasn't aware.

In her book *Nobody, Nowhere: The Extraordinary Autobiography of an Autistic,* Donna Williams, an autistic adult, describes tiny spots, she called them stars, that surrounded her bed. She later learned that these spots were actually air particles that she could see with her hypersensitive vision.[3]

Does Benjamin also perceive something that we can't see, I wondered.

One bright morning, we took a trip on the light rail train near our home. Benjamin had a habit of running off the train at our stop and racing to the front of the train until he stood even with the first set of train wheels. He would stare at the wheels until the train continued on its path. Benjamin would begin "stimming" as the train departed, and continue until he could no longer see the wheels, then watch passively until the second set of wheels passed, when he would engage in "stimming" again. After the train passed, he would gaze out briefly at the tracks where the train had just passed. We had observed him doing this hundreds of times, but had no idea why he did this. My husband and I were discussing this fact when my six-year-old daughter offered her thoughts.

"I know why he's staring at the tracks," my daughter commented, as we watched Benjamin staring at the back of the train as it continued down its path.

"Why?" I asked.

"He's seeing the purple light that runs in a thin line on the tracks," she replied.

"You see purple light on the tracks?" I asked.

"Yes," she replied casually.

"Do you see anything near the train's wheels?" I asked.

"Yes, just the same purple light, but it's going in a circle around the wheels."

"Do you see any light on the tracks here?" I asked, pointing at the tracks right where we were standing.

"No. The light follows right behind the train and just a little ways behind it," she replied matter of factly.

"Well, there you have it," my husband replied. "You just never know what a family outing might bring."

Trains are fascinating objects for many autistic children. Perhaps if we saw as they do, they would be fascinating to us as well.

A few months later, Karis drew a picture of the train, showing what the train wheels looked like to her. The picture showed purple surrounding the wheels of the train, with a band of blue a short distance from the purple. What was startling about the picture wasn't the wheels, which were as she described them, but what she drew on top of the train. The light rail train is an electric powered train that operates by taking electricity from an overhead cable. Metal bars run from the top of the train car to the wire, bringing electric current into the structure. Karis drew a field of pink around this structure, which carries the electricity to the train (see figure 1, color section). Not having any understanding of how the train operated, she unwittingly demonstrated that she was seeing a color associated with the electric field of the train. What is going on here, I wondered. How can my daughter perceive electricity in full color?

Once, Benjamin became very uncomfortable with a drawing on one of his therapist's walls. It was a drawing of a man with acupuncture points indicated on the body. It was not particularly graphic, in that it was just a line drawing of a man. The therapist had much more graphic drawings positioned directly beside this drawing. Benjamin refused to enter the treatment room until the drawing was removed. Why did he consistently react negatively to this drawing, so much so that he continued to make sure that it had been removed each time before entering the treatment room? Why did he consistently "stim" when looking at children's art or art by famous artists, yet react so adversely to this drawing? Why would he completely ignore the art of lesser-known artists? What was he seeing that we didn't?

Benjamin experienced great difficulty with trips to the airport. He began to engage in his "forced running" behavior in order to handle the stimulation. He had to be allowed to run, or he would scream. I have met two men who have characteristics similar to Benjamin, but neither one is considered autistic. These two men provided invaluable insight on some of Benjamin's more unique behaviors. They are both very sensitive and perceive subtle energies of which most people are unaware. One man, although he earns a good living for his family, is unable to find his way home from the neighborhood grocery store or to operate an automobile. When asked why airports and airplanes posed such a challenge for Benjamin, he replied that he, too, hated airports and traveling by airplane. He explained that airplanes and airports are packed full of electronics and radio wave frequencies, not to mention people and their corresponding emotions. He is able physically to feel these energy fields, and they make him extremely uncomfortable. He explained that during airplane flights, his perceptions are "speeded up" to such a degree that he becomes quite disoriented.

On my next airplane trip, I decided to go into a meditative state to try and feel what Benjamin felt while on an airplane. The first sensation I felt was one of extreme uneasiness in the pit of my stomach. I saw a bright flash of yellow-white light, which I could only describe as something between a small lightning bolt and static electricity. I felt these jolts periodically coursing through my body. The feeling was like being propelled through wide, thin sheets of static electricity. Upon opening my eyes, I saw that my vision was very unsteady. Any turbulence greatly increased the unpleasant sensations. No wonder Benjamin needs a good distraction on airplanes, I thought.

On that same occasion, I had a four-hour layover in the Dallas/Fort Worth airport and decided to go into a meditative state to see if I could feel what Benjamin was feeling when he was in an airport. At first I felt a slight inward pressure in my head. My body began to feel constricted, yet I felt lightheaded. I could hear the creaking of the knees as people passed in the aisle in front of me. I felt the slap of each step on the tile floor echoing in my head. The rustling of a trash bag reverberated in my head. It was a symphony of chaos. Colors were very vivid. I had a difficult time controlling my body as the energy of every movement physically slammed back and forth in my body. The glare of a bald man's head caught my attention, and I longed to continue staring at it. I felt the energy of a cell phone as its holder walked past me. As it passed, I immediately became aware of all other cell phone users, as they were simultaneously brought into my conscious awareness. A slight chill rolled down my spine. Everyone's eyes met mine. Why was that, I wondered.

A neon tube of colored light ran along a wall. I could barely take my eyes from it to write notes in my journal. A bright white and a purplish blue more intense than any I had ever seen was alternating with a brick red color. Although my overall state was dreamlike and comfortable, suddenly I was uncomfortable sitting in the chair, as I perceived a soup of sound and sleepiness. A janitor walked by and I felt a stabbing sensation in my throat area. The pain passed through me as he passed. I sensed that it was caused by his small two-way radio. I saw a woman's long braid across the room, and I wanted to inspect the weave of her hair more closely. The braid moved and twisted as she turned her head.

I could feel the subtle, natural rhythms of my body. As soon as I focused on something, the room seemed to close in around it. Behind me, lights flickered, and it startled and panicked me. I felt a million miles away, yet intensely focused on wherever my gaze fell. I recoiled as a worker with a carpet sweeper swept in front of me, and it felt like he was dragging the sweeper across the surface of my skin in short, brisk strokes. A man walking by carried a plate of food, and it glistened in the light. A ringing phone remained unanswered and created great tension in my body. I suppressed the urge to run and get away from it. The pressure in my head increased, and I felt as if I was on the verge of panic. My stomach tightened and my breathing was shallow.

As I slowly brought myself back to normal awareness, I had a much greater understanding and empathy for my son in this situation. I don't know how I was able to perceive as he did, but I knew that what I perceived at the airport that day was very different from anything I had ever perceived before. I knew that I was on to something when I read the words of Donna Williams describing the normal state of mind of her world. She describes being in a hypnotic state where she could "grasp the depth of the simplest of things; everything was reduced to colors, rhythms, and sensations."[4] Her words were the perfect description of my airport experience.

Benjamin, like most autistic children, didn't have any understanding of linear concepts. He did much better with pictures, which allowed him to form a mental picture of a situation, rather than a verbal one.

He had no concept of waiting in lines. He would rush to the front of the line, totally focused on whatever drew his attention there. The only way to handle this situation was to have plenty of items to distract him with, but these tactics were seldom successful for long. Most of the time he would began screaming and kicking, and we would have to leave.

Video arcades caused Benjamin to revert into his sideways looking and running behavior. The stimulation was simply too much for his body to handle. He would become completely out of control. Large crowds produced the same effect. He simply shut down and began screaming. Why do these situations cause him such great physical and emotional discomfort, I wondered.

5 The Natural Medicine Treatments

Our birth is but a sleep and a forgetting,
The soul that rises with us—our life's star
Has had elsewhere its setting
And cometh from afar.
Not in entire forgetfulness
And not in utter nakedness
But trailing clouds of glory do we come
From God who is our home.

—*William Wordsworth*

I had no way of knowing that Benjamin's milk allergy was a blessing. I went to the local health food store shortly after Benjamin's first birthday, looking for a suitable milk substitute for him to drink. As luck would have it, a good friend was in the store that day. We were discussing the possibilities when a woman approached. She apologized for eavesdropping, and told of her own experience with very severe food allergies. Handing me a folded piece of paper with the name of a person in Houston, she explained that this therapist had somehow cured her food allergies with a treatment called CranioSacral Therapy. My friend knew of some therapists in our town who were trained in that therapy, so I called and made an appointment that day.

On Benjamin's first appointment, I wondered if I had made a mistake. He cried almost the entire hour. The therapist, with a very light touch, put her hands on various parts of Ben's body. Ben seemed to be in agony, although his reaction was much more severe than simply being touched by a stranger seemed to warrant. He seemed to be someplace very far away, looking right through me, unaware that I was there, willing to comfort him.

"Benjamin is not allowing me to work on the milk allergy," the therapist said, pausing hesitantly. "I'm finding a hip problem, and he wants me to correct it first," she continued.

Yeah, right. I thought. So much for keeping an open mind, I chided myself.

"The hip problem occurred during his birth. His delivery was very fast, wasn't it?" she asked.

"Yes, he was born very quickly," I replied, wondering how she could have known that.

As she concluded the treatment, she commented, "Benjamin might act strangely after the therapy. Just be aware that he may have some unusual behavior after the treatment."

Okay, I thought, only half listening. I was wondering if I was a bad mother for letting my child cry for an hour without stopping the treatment.

I soon realized that the therapist's comment about Benjamin having unusual behavior was an understatement. When Benjamin awoke from his nap later that day, he began wailing and crying and holding his hip in the exact location that the therapist had treated that morning. Attempts to hold him or console him were pointless. I laid him back down, as he appeared to be in a trance, crying in agony, unaware of my presence. The episode lasted a full 15 minutes, then his demeanor abruptly changed. He sat up, looked around the room as if he had just woken from his nap, wide-eyed and ready to play. Thank goodness the therapist had warned me about the strange behavior. I probably would have rushed him to the emergency room, thinking he was having an appendicitis attack.

He repeated this scenario several times over the next few days, including once when my husband was home, and another time when my mother was caring for him. I was glad to have witnesses. Otherwise, I might have feared that I was losing my mind. What was happening? I had no frame of reference when it came to the things that I was seeing my one-year-old child do. As Benjamin was so young, I knew that he should not be influenced by the therapist or by her expectations, yet he appeared to be working through the same injury she had discovered, and he was doing it when he wasn't even fully awake. When Benjamin began the therapy, he was just under 13 months old and had not even attempted to walk. Within a few days of the therapy, he began walking and then running.

I grew up in a traditional family setting. My father worked and my mother stayed at home with her three daughters until we reached school age. For many years, our illnesses were treated with conventional medicine by a wonderful tender-hearted physician who would have to leave the room when one of us cried. At the first sign of illness, we were whisked off to his crowded waiting room with all the other ill people who needed a good dose of his compassion. I was unaware of any other forms of treatment, except for a handful of visits to a chiropractor when I was a teenager, when stubborn back and neck pain would not resolve itself. Benjamin's experience was completely foreign to me, but I knew that something was happening, and nothing in my life experiences up until that point could offer any insight as to what that something might be.

Due to Benjamin's violent reactions to milk, I still religiously kept him away from milk and dairy products, even though he was undergoing therapy. A few months later, while checking out at a local store, I failed to notice some cheese puff samples beside the cash register.

"Oh my God," I gasped, as I watched the fat little orange cheese puff disappear into Benjamin's mouth. Clenching his teeth behind a wide satisfied grin, Benjamin began quickly chewing the cheese puff. The clerk stared at me like I was from Mars as I leaned Benjamin backward, shoving my finger into his mouth, trying to pry open his teeth. He clenched his teeth tightly together. It was no use. I stood paralyzed at the checkout counter, trying to remember if I had put one of his epinephrine injectors in my purse, wondering if I could actually shove a needle into Benjamin's thigh.

Thirty seconds, and no reaction, one minute and no projectile vomiting. Maybe it wasn't going to happen this time. I tried not to think about his doctor's comment about his dropping dead on the school cafeteria floor, but the pictures were already flashing into my mind. I waited for what seemed like hours, as the people in line behind me wondered if the psychotic lunatic in front of them was ever going to leave. Benjamin grinned an openmouthed smile. The cheese puff was gone, and he was quite proud of himself. To my amazement, he had no reaction. I shakily scooped him up and carried him to the parking lot, almost afraid to believe what I had witnessed.

I decided that I'd better begin educating myself about Cranio-Sacral Therapy. I scheduled an appointment for myself and began questioning the therapist to learn more about how the therapy worked. She gave me a copy of *Your Inner Physician and You* by Dr. John E. Upledger.[1] I signed up for a beginning course to learn the therapy so that I could work with Benjamin at home. I learned that Cranio-Sacral Therapy was developed by an osteopathic physician, John E. Upledger, following extensive scientific studies at Michigan State University, where he served as a clinical researcher and professor of biomechanics.

The therapy is a gentle, hands-on method of evaluating and enhancing the functioning of a physiological body system called the craniosacral system, which is comprised of the membranes and cerebrospinal fluid that surround and protect the brain and spinal cord. Using a soft touch, generally no greater than the weight of a nickel, practitioners release restrictions in the craniosacral system to improve the functioning of the central nervous system. The therapy complements the body's own natural healing processes and bolsters resistance to disease. What I didn't know at that time was that CranioSacral Therapy was effective treatment for his undiagnosed autism spectrum disorder. I believe that Benjamin's symptoms, particularly those involving his physical body, would have been much more severe if he hadn't received CranioSacral Therapy from the time he was one year old.

At my own therapy sessions, I began to feel sensations in my body that I had never felt before. My chronic back pain diminished and my overall general health improved. The therapist located traumas to my body that I had long ago forgotten. She discovered a trauma from a blunt force striking me between my shoulders. When I was a teenager, I had been hit in the back by a kicked football at a high school football game. My body had remembered the injury, both physically and emotionally, long after my mind had let it slip away.

She found the injury to my legs from a car accident. The therapist was unaware that I had been suffering from leg pain. During a side impact collision, my legs hit the center console of the car. I remembered thinking at the time that the force at which my legs struck the console must have broken them, but they appeared unharmed, except for a slight soreness. The therapist knew that one leg had the trauma to the outside of the leg and the other one to the inside of the leg. Somehow, the therapist was able to tap into my body's history. She was aware of very specific information that was of an unusual nature. Neither injury had required medical treatment when it occurred, yet each was having long-term negative effects on my body. Both areas of my body have remained pain-free since the treatments.

In *The Natural Medicine Guide to Autism,* Stephanie Marohn outlines in detail cranial osteopathy's role in resolving birth trauma in autistic children, and how SomatoEmotional Release assists the body in discharging the stored emotions that result from trauma and block the body's energy flow, resulting in physical dysfunction.[2] Benjamin's treatments involved both therapies. His emotional episodes after his treatments, when he was crying and appeared to be in a trance, were spontaneous SomatoEmotional Release that continued to help him work through trauma.

I began to share these experiences in my weekly meditation classes. My meditation teacher met a man while at a retreat and wanted to bring him to our town to teach his own method of body healing. He was a physical therapist trained in CranioSacral Therapy, but he practiced extensively in many areas of the healing arts. He specialized in teaching a person to connect with his own unique healing force in order to heal himself. To me, this sounded exactly like what Benjamin and I were experiencing in our therapy sessions. I signed up to take the class and offered to let the teacher stay in our home during the course of the class.

In a synchronistic turn of good fortune, the teacher arrived to teach the class the day after we received Benjamin's official diagnosis. He offered to assess Benjamin and concluded that some of the immunizations Benjamin had received were causing many of the difficulties that he was experiencing. He treated Benjamin that evening while he was asleep, using LEAP (Learning Enhancement Advanced Program) techniques.[3] As he treated Benjamin, I went into the kitchen to fix the therapist something to drink. As I poured the drink into a glass, I suddenly began choking. I had the sensation that the tissues in my throat were swelling, not allowing me to take a breath. It took several minutes for the sensation to subside and for my breathing to return to normal.

When I returned to the living room where the therapist was treating Benjamin, he explained that I was probably feeling the same sensations that Benjamin felt after receiving the particular immunization that he was balancing in Benjamin's system. He explained further that the immunization had been particularly hard on Benjamin's system. I didn't really know what to think of this statement at the time, but I could not explain why I would suddenly begin choking for no apparent reason. I was not eating or drinking anything when it occurred, and I could not ever remember feeling similar sensations before that day. It was my first conscious experience with clairsentience, feeling the emotional and physical responses that another person is feeling.

LEAP, the technique used by the therapist to balance Benjamin's immunizations, was developed by Dr. Charles T. Krebs at Melbourne Applied Physiology in Australia. The therapy resolves stressed areas of the brain using kinesiology and acupressure techniques. The program helps to repattern brain activity around problem areas. The therapy itself is interesting to observe. The therapist touches specific areas of the patient's body and actually uses his own body for storing information.

I knew that some people believed that immunizations had been the cause, or at least a factor in the progression of their child's autistic symptoms. I had formed no opinion on this, until Benjamin woke up the next morning. He got up, stood in the living room like he was trying to get his bearings, and then looked directly into the therapist's face. Then, he ran to the back door and opened it. He began to run in circles looking sideways, but something caught his eye. The therapist, my husband, and I watched as Benjamin stopped abruptly, bending down toward a group of flowers. Tears poured down my cheeks as he noticed and then touched a flower for the first time. He focused his attention on the flower for about 30 seconds. In the hundreds of times Benjamin had run in the backyard in the past, he had never noticed a flower before that day.

As the therapist began to teach the course that he had developed, I realized that his healing system involved assessing restrictions in the body's electromagnetic field, commonly called the aura. The healing is accomplished on four levels: the physical body, the emotional body, the mental body, and the spiritual body. The levels surround the body in all directions and are located from four to 26 inches from the physical body. The system also assesses the chakras, which are the pathways for the body's life-force energy. I knew that the presence of chakras in the energy field was well documented in the Eastern yogic tradition. Although by that time I had met several people who claimed to be able to see the human auric field, the therapist could not but had learned to feel the differences with his hands by studying extensively with Dan Friesen, a Canadian spiritual healer who could see auras. I was delighted to learn that I could feel the differences and locate restrictions on the various levels of the energy field.

When I returned home that evening, Benjamin's gaze locked onto me from across the room. He ran across the room toward me, staring intently with his attention focused near the top of my head. He reached out with a flat palm, extending his arm about two feet from my head, and slowly lowered his hand until he physically touched my head. In class earlier that day, we had discovered that this exact area of my head had the most severe restriction in my auric field. As we were just learning to locate these restrictions, it had not yet been healed. The therapist entered the room just in time to see Benjamin make a beeline toward me. Again, I had a witness. Benjamin could see what I had just learned to feel!

I realized that I had seen Benjamin demonstrate this behavior once before. Several months previously, I was practicing CranioSacral Therapy on a friend with Alzheimer-type symptoms when Benjamin ran into the room. Circling the treatment table, he ran looking sideways, as was his custom at that time. As my friend lay supine on the table, something caught Benjamin's attention. Stopping abruptly, he focused intently on an area above my friend's head. Reaching up as high as he could with his left hand in a flattened palm, he positioned his hand directly above my friend's left eye. Like a child playing with the light shining through a prism, he "stimmed" as he slowly lowered his hand until it was scarcely an inch above my friend's left eye. Then, he quickly removed his hand and ran out of the room. I did not give it any more thought until my friend's wife called me later that day.

"Keli, what did you do to my husband?" she asked.

"Why?" I asked hesitantly.

"Because he is acting just like his old self. His head seems clear. This is the best he's been in years," she said excitedly.

"I just did CranioSacral Therapy, exactly as I've done before, except that Benjamin seemed to see something directly above John's eye."

"Maybe he did something to John," she joked.

My friend had been asleep while Benjamin was in the room, but he mentioned before he left that day that he had suffered a concussion while playing football in high school. This friend, a physical therapist, had attended the healing class that day, and we realized that Benjamin had located his worst restriction, which was positioned directly above his left eye!

What exactly was an aura, and why could Benjamin see it when so many people, myself included, could not? Not content with esoteric explanations, I began searching for more concrete, scientific information about what he was seeing.

Persons who are able to see auras report seeing an energy field, seen as a light, surrounding all living things. In 1729, Sir Isaac Newton spoke of this light and described it as excitable, exhibiting characteristics of motion, repulsion, and attraction. In the 1930s Dr. Harold Burr found these fields exist around people, animals, trees, plants, seeds, eggs, and even slime molds. He began over 40 years of scientific research on these fields and theorized that they were responsible for the body's capacity for cell regeneration and tended to serve as a template that allowed new cells to behave exactly like the cells they replaced. He believed that this field could give advance warning of a dysfunction in the body, even before actual physical symptoms manifested.

In *Wheels of Light*, Rosalyn L. Bruyere states that "[A] healer can detect these electrodynamic or energy inconsistencies through touch or sight." She maintains that with such forewarning, "preventive action, whether a specific medical or psychological process or a rebalancing of energies through healing, may then be taken."[4]

She points to the 20 years of research by Dr. Robert Becker as establishing the relationship between regeneration and electrical currents in living things and believes "this electromagnetic flow also provides cells with the appropriate electrical environment to either sustain health within an uninjured cell or stimulate healing in a damaged cell." This flow is the "passageway utilized by healers when they channel energy into a client to bring about healing."[5] She concludes that the auric field, which is created and controlled by the chakras, is really a metaphor for life. The aura actually mirrors the flow of a person's life and is life itself.

Persons who are able to see these energies and auric fields are called clairvoyant. Bruyere theorizes that people who possess this ability may be speeding up the normal process of visual perception.[6] Maybe this was how Benjamin was able to see the body's energy field. I still wanted more concrete information about how this all worked. Sure, I really couldn't deny that he was seeing something, and I believe that at least some other autistic children experience this phenomenon, too.

I once saw one of Benjamin's classmates "stimming" by moving his fingers in front of his eyes. He was holding his hands out in front of his face, with his fingers pointing inward toward each other, just a few inches apart. He was rocking back and forth, moving his fingers. What I noticed at the time was that he wasn't looking at his fingers; he was looking intently at the space directly in front of him, between his fingers as he moved them, as if there were some amazing phenomenon occurring there.

Since then, I have discovered that there are secondary chakras that extend out from each finger. Secondary chakras are smaller vortices that exist primarily wherever there is a joint in the body, where bone touches bone. To people who see auras, they appear as little cyclones, whirling vortexes of energy with each finger emanating a different color, either red, green, blue, or violet (see figure 2, color section). What a wonderful and fascinating sight the movement of all that color and energy would be, if one could see it.

Often, Benjamin "stims" when looking at a person's hip, or at the bottom of the feet, both of which are locations of secondary chakras. I discovered that there was a long history of various traditions that recognized the auric field and the chakras as valid systems, but I still had many questions about how all of this worked. Little did I know that I would have to delve into the world of physics in order to get some answers.

I didn't have to go far to find experts in the field. Sitting across from me at my weekly meditation sessions were two physicists who were professors at a large university. Dr. Robert Unterberger retired after teaching electromagnetic resonance at a major university for more than 25 years. We began informal discussions about how and why this might all be occurring. I knew I had to understand energy at its simplest levels in order to begin to understand what was happening with Benjamin. The other dear friend, Dr. Ronald Bryan, began methodically and patiently teaching me about physics, helping me to grasp what is currently believed about the interplay between the forces of nature. When I delved into the world of modern physics, I discovered that physical matter is not what our physical senses perceive it to be.

When Dr. W. Brugh Joy was practicing internal medicine in Los Angeles, he contracted a life-threatening disease that culminated in an illuminating meditation, which caused him to abruptly give up his medical practice. Six weeks later he discovered that his illness was completely cured. He explains our perception of matter in relationship to the reality of physics in his book *Joy's Way:*

> [M]atter is not what our physical senses report it as being. Our senses tell us that our bodies are solid, "real" objects encased in a solid, "real" skin covering. These "realities" are what we experience as our physical selves. We are unaware of our bodies' activities at the cellular level, let alone the molecular and atomic levels, and to approach the subatomic levels and relate them to our own form and structure is mostly intellectual ideation and not in any way experiential.[7]

He explains the progression in our understanding of the human body as follows:

> [A]wareness of the human body has progressed from the level of gross form and structure, to the level of the organ systems, to the cellular level, to the molecular level, to the submolecular level and finally to atomic and subatomic levels.

On these latter levels we don't find matter—we find only swirling or oscillating fields of energy, and between these observable energy interactions we find an unbelievable amount of what appears to be nothingness. The truth is that our bodies—like all "matter"—are composed of a great deal of nothingness and a smidgen of matter or energy interaction. An atomic nucleus and its electrons are both energies, and the distance between them, relative to their sizes, is in proportion to the distance between the sun and the earth. There is a vast amount of nothingness.[8]

There is evidence that this "nothingness" is actually the area of electromagnetic field activity. While attending a CranioSacral Therapy class, I picked up a copy of *Infinite Mind: Science of the Human Vibrations of Consciousness,* by Dr. Valerie V. Hunt. From her laboratory at UCLA, Dr. Hunt developed a comprehensive human energy field model based on her 25 years of electronic field research. She explains that the body's electrical activity is essential for life. Many researchers have sought the essence of life in the heart, muscles, nerve electricity, and biochemistry of the human body. With recent discoveries proving that "all cells, even subatomic particles, contain tiny electrical elements, there is a growing belief that life is electromagnetic and cannot be explained by mechanical or biochemical means."[9]

Dr. Hunt explains that there are two primary electrical systems in the physical body:

One is the well-known alternative electric current of the nervous system—the brain, neurons, and the nerves—which causes muscle contraction, nerve transmission, glandular secretion, and sensation. The other is a newly discovered electromagnetic system probably emanating from atoms and cells. This energy has been called an aura, though I prefer to describe it as an energy field.

The pool of electromagnetic energy around an object or a person allows energy exchange. This corona, invisible to most people, is seen at times as a halo or light-colored mist around a living body. Although composed of the same electrons as inert substances, the human field absorbs and throws off energy dynamically. It interacts with and influences matter, whereas fields associated with inert matter react passively.[10]

She discovered that the energy field was unique, in that it was continuous, while "the other body electric recordings of heart, brain, and muscle are off-and-on signals: a muscle contraction is followed by muscle relaxation; a heartbeat is followed by a quiet rest period; and a brain wave is followed by lesser action."[11]

Physics, the source of all information about the universe, tells us that all matter, whether inert or living matter, is composed of atoms. In each atom, electrons spin around a nucleus, throwing off some electrons. Free electrons, from living things, human-made objects, or the natural physical environment, rush in to balance this unstable state.

The Natural Medicine Guide to Autism, quoting Dr. Dietrich Klinghart, M.D., Ph.D., based in Bellevue, Washington, explains the body's energetic field in terms of the traffic of information in the nervous system:

> Eighty percent of the messages are going up to the brain (from the body), and twenty percent of the messages go down from the brain (to the body). The nerve currents moving up and down generate a magnetic field that goes out into space, creating an electromagnetic field around the body that interacts with other fields.[12]

It appeared that existence of the human auric field has been scientifically verified. I had no idea at the time that this was just the beginning of my understanding as to what was happening with Benjamin.

As I was studying the more unusual aspects of Benjamin's condition, I was simultaneously researching any existing treatments that seemed to increase the comfort level of autistic children. A friend gave me a copy of *Unraveling the Mystery of Autism and Pervasive Developmental Disorder* by Karyn Seroussi. I was particularly interested in the dietary interventions the author presented. Due to Benjamin's milk allergy, he was already on a casein-free diet. I decided to try a treatment for overgrowth of intestinal yeast *(Candida)*. Because the recommended drug was nonsystemic, not absorbed into the blood-stream, I felt that it was unlikely to harm Benjamin's sensitive system, but I needed a doctor's prescription.

I mentioned the dietary interventions and immunization theo-ries at Benjamin's next doctor's appointment. The doctor summarily dismissed dietary interventions as "unnecessary" and the immuniza-tion theory as "baseless." Based on the doctor's reaction, I couldn't bring myself to ask for a prescription for nystatin, which was the rec-ommended drug for the yeast treatment. Instead, a sympathetic and open-minded dentist friend prescribed it for Benjamin. It had to be special ordered in powdered form, since all prepared nystatin treat-ments contain large amounts of sugar to cover its unpleasant taste. Unfortunately, sugar feeds the yeast, which defeats the purpose of the treatment, which is to starve the yeast growth.

I dissolved the powdered, sugar-free nystatin powder in water and religiously administered the bitter-tasting liquid using a small needle-less syringe into Benjamin's mouth several times each day over the course of a week. The administration of the nystatin was trau-matic, but we immediately noticed an improvement in his behavior. The most noticeable difference was the evidence in his diaper. His stool was normally yellowish in color and soft in its consistency. After the course of treatment, his stool became normal and has remained normal with no additional treatment.

I found that there is some evidence that the intestinal yeast prob-lem may be caused by the measles-mumps-rubella vaccine. In *The Natural Medicine Guide to Autism,* Stephanie Marohn cites testimony by Dr. Andrew Wakefield before the U.S. Congressional Oversight Committee on Government Reform:

> Rather than having parental reports alone of a temporal association between MMR exposure and developmental regression, there is now definitive evidence of a novel and specific pathology in the intestine of children with ASD (autistic spectrum disorder) that is associated with the pres-ence of measles virus. In association with the findings of Kawashima et al., of measles virus in the peripheral blood of some children with ASD, it is no longer correct or acceptable

to state that there is no evidence of an association between MMR and this syndrome. In light of this and in view of the acknowledged lack of adequate safety studies on the MMR vaccine, the case for making MMR vaccination either mandatory or the exclusive mode of protection against measles, mumps and rubella is, in my opinion, difficult to justify. Parents should be given an informed choice of vaccination strategy, including the provision of single vaccines.[13]

I was stunned when I remembered that Benjamin received not only his MMR vaccine, but the only other live-virus vaccine routinely administered to children, the Varicella (chicken pox) vaccine, on the same day, just shy of his first birthday, when he yelled "Let's go!" as we were leaving his doctor's office. Four live viruses assaulted his little body and immune system on the same day! How could it be coincidence that Benjamin spoke using two words correctly for the first time on that day, but subsequently lost that ability for more than two years?

Another suggestion I tried was to supplement Benjamin with DMG, a naturally occurring amino acid. I attempted to give Benjamin various vitamins that were recommended in Seroussi's book, but he seemed to be able to taste any differences in the liquids I tried to mask them in, and refused to take them.

I began to research the connection between learning disabilities and vaccinations. I discovered a wonderful book, *What Your Doctor May Not Tell You About Children's Vaccinations,* by Stephanie Cave, M.D. The book lists one ingredient in vaccines, thimerosal, which is a substance that contains nearly 50 percent ethylmercury, a form of mercury. I had known almost 20 years before that I was extremely allergic to thimerosal. The substance was used as a preservative in many eye care products, including contact lens solutions. A large proportion of the population suffered ill effects, and within a short time, it was removed from many eye care products. I was stunned that a substance that had been known for 20 years to cause such severe adverse reactions would be removed from many eye care products, but not from children's vaccinations!

According to Dr. Cave's research, the amount of mercury in immunizations was discovered almost by accident. In 1997, Frank Pallone, a New Jersey congressman, was concerned about the amount of mercury people could be ingesting in their food and drugs. He wrote an amendment to a Food and Drug Administration bill asking the FDA to "compile a list of drugs and foods that contain intentionally introduced mercury compounds and [to] provide a quantitative and qualitative analysis of the mercury compounds in the list." The resulting list ended up "inciting fear among parents, concern among researchers, and protests from manufacturers. It was an investigation that led to the realization that mercury—a known toxic substance that can cause behavioral problems, learning disorders, and many other medical conditions—was being injected into infants and young children under the guise of safe, government-sanctioned, routine vaccinations."[14]

The following excerpt from the book frightened both the mother in me, and the attorney in me:

The Mercury/Thimerosal-Autism Connection

Between 1991 and 1999 the United States embarked on what might be labeled a bold, ill-planned experiment: the recommended vaccination of newborns with the hepatitis B vaccine. This vaccine contained 12.5 micrograms of mercury (thimerosal), which is more than 25 times the EPA "safe level" of 0.1 microgram per kilogram of body weight per day. This toxic dose was followed by not one but two more doses: one at one to two months and another at six months of age. In addition, infants and children were also given four doses of mercury-containing HiB at two, four, six, and 12 to 15 months of age: plus four doses of mercury-containing DTP at two, four, six, and 12 to 18 months of age. By the age of six months, vaccinated children had received 187.5 mcg of mercury—a poison that accumulated in their bodies because production of the bile, which helps clear toxins from the body, is not developed in children less than four to six months of age.

When mercury can't get out of the body, it travels to the brain, changes into inorganic mercury, clings to brain tissue, and damages the nervous system. Mercury doesn't just cling to any part of the brain; it goes exactly to those areas involved in autism: the cerebellum, amygdala, and hippocampus. The

cerebellum is involved in the execution of balance and movement, such as walking and running, and the smooth movements of the eye; the amygdala controls emotional
processing; and the hippocampus is involved in the forma-
tion, sorting, and storage of memory.[15]

Dr. David Baskin, a neurological surgery professor at Baylor
College of Medicine in Houston, Texas, testified before the U.S.
Congressional Oversight Committee on Government Reform that we
should "make no mistake there is an intent to put a preservative in
these vaccines to prevent the growth of microorganisms [which] has
gone awry because the preservative that was used ended up being a
poison."[16] He continued by saying that "there is no debate in the scientific literature that mercury is a potent neurotoxin," and that this
information had been known since the late 1890s. He pointed out
that thimerosal was first placed in vaccines in the late 1930s, and
three years later, Leo Kanner first described the syndrome of autism.
In *The Natural Medicine Guide to Autism,* Stephanie Marohn outlines many of the same concerns. She quotes Dr. Tim O'Shea who
describes three particular days as "spectacularly toxic" for infants:

> Shortly after birth when the baby receives the hepatitis B
> vaccine, which contains 12 mcg of mercury (30 times the
> official safe level); at four months when the infant receives
> the DtaP and HiB, with a total of 50 mcg of mercury (60
> times the safe level), on the same day; and at six months
> when the child receives Hep B and polio on the same day,
> with 62.5 mcg of mercury (78 times the safe level).[17]

In Dr. Cave's book and in Stephanie Marohn's book, each author
presents a chart that compares the characteristics of autism and mercury poisoning.[18] The similarities are staggering. I also learned that
the hepatitis B vaccine, administered to Benjamin on his first day of
life, is the most controversial. People who are at risk to this disease
are intravenous drug users, homosexual men, prostitutes, individuals
with multiple sexual partners, health-care workers who handle needles or blood, individuals who live in a household in which someone
has hepatitis B, employees and inmates of correctional institutions,

and infants born to mothers who have hepatitis B.[19] Less than one percent of infants fall into the risk category, being born to mothers who have hepatitis B.

The decision was made in 1991 to give the vaccination to all newborns, even though the vast majority of them are in no danger of contracting the disease. This decision was made because too few of the adults in the high-risk groups were being immunized.

Bonnie S. Dunbar, Ph.D., a professor at Baylor College of Medicine and a pioneer in vaccine research, believes that the hepatitis B vaccine is "a serious, perhaps even deadly, threat to a portion of the population that may have a genetic makeup that makes them react negatively to the vaccine."[20] Her research suggests Caucasians of northern European descent may be at higher risk of reacting to the vaccine. Benjamin, being of Norwegian descent, falls within this category. Rather than the mass immunization of all infants, it would be easier, less expensive, and much safer to screen pregnant women for hepatitis B and immunize the less than one percent of infants who are actually at risk for the disease. Where was logic and reason when it came to protecting our children, I wondered.

We found Behice Kutay, a wonderful therapist in Austin trained in LEAP therapy, CranioSacral Therapy, Lymph Drainage therapy, and many other healing techniques, who continued Benjamin's treatments. Lymph Drainage therapy focuses on the functioning of the body's lymphatic system, and was developed by Bruno Chikly, M.D., a French physician.[21] A properly functioning lymphatic system drains fluids, detoxifies and regenerates tissues, filters out toxins and foreign substances, and helps maintain a healthy immune system. If lymph circulation stagnates, toxins accumulate and compromise cellular functions, opening a pathway to physical ailments. I began taking Benjamin on weekly two-hour trips to Austin for his therapy sessions.

Using LEAP techniques, Behice began methodically balancing the effects of each immunization he had received. She balanced Benjamin for anything that appeared to put him under physical or emotional stress. With a muscle response testing technique, she determined whether there was stress.

Muscle response testing is a simple test to determine good or bad electromagnetic field interaction of a single food, medication, substance, or immunization. The substance is placed in the energy field of the patient, then an applied kinesiological manual testing of the muscle strength of the arm is performed. If the muscles test strong to downward pressure on the arm, the field interaction is positive and that substance is not harmful to the person. If the muscles become weakened and the arm cannot resist pressure, the field interaction is poor and the substance should be avoided.

In *Energy Medicine*, Donna Eden explains the biological basis for muscle response, or energy testing. She describes the nervous system of the human body as a "phenomenally sensitive 37-mile-long antenna that reverberates to the subtle and not-so-subtle energies of the world in which you live."[22] She maintains that everything from the food you eat to the people you encounter carries its own frequency and impacts the nervous system, with the human body resonating to some vibrations and tensing against others, which is reflected by the resistance in the muscle used for the test.

Dr. Valerie Hunt performed a simple test to determine the immediate effects of fabrics, chemicals, and electromagnetic radiation on the strength of muscle.[23] Four volunteers were selected, and each person was brought separately into an area that was contaminated by an operating television, microwave oven, computers, and fluorescent lights. They were dressed in synthetic fiber and placed on a synthetic rug. The atmosphere was further contaminated by the introduction of paint remover, ammonia, bleach, and fingernail polish remover; hairspray and aerosol air freshener were also sprayed in the environment. The shoulder muscle of each person was tested using a Cibex computerized dynamometer that flashed the actual foot pounds that those muscles could generate before, during, and after contamination. In each instance, the strength of the muscles dropped one-quarter to one-half during contamination.

When the contaminated field was blown out using fans, the muscle strength returned but not to the pretest level. When a tape of the actual recordings of the sound of the human aura, a coherent field, was played, the muscle strength increased to a higher foot poundage than was generated during the pretest.

The success of LEAP therapy techniques has affirmed the benefits of muscle response testing. Benjamin was balanced for food allergies, airborne allergies, electromagnetic radiation, even for family members and teachers! He was balanced several more times for each immunization he received that continued to affect his field negatively. I began to notice that if Benjamin were ill before his therapy treatments, he would improve greatly after the therapy, usually fully recovering from the illness by the next day.

Soon, I had a rare opportunity to test conventional antibiotic therapy against his natural medicine therapies. Benjamin had come down with another case of croup. I had given him a full ten-day course of an oral antibiotic. He improved somewhat physically, but by the eleventh day, he had become very ill again and his cough was more severe than before. I was exasperated that I had endured 11 days of his tantrums and behavior problems, only to see the illness recur. When I called his pediatrician's office and scheduled the earliest appointment available for that afternoon, the nurse mentioned that some children with this condition were not responding to antibiotics, and the croup would often progress into pneumonia.

I immediately called Behice, who agreed to clear her calendar in order to treat Benjamin before his doctor's appointment. My mother agreed to accompany us to Austin. Benjamin was lethargic and pale, and I was afraid that he might become more ill during the trip and I might need her help. We loaded Benjamin into our van, and set out for the trip to Austin. Benjamin's appetite had dropped off during his illness. When we passed the familiar golden arches where we always stopped to get Benjamin's favorite french fries, he didn't protest.

Upon our arrival at the therapist's office, she began doing Lymph Drainage therapy on Benjamin's chest area. He was unusually still and cooperative. He simply didn't have the energy to fidget. She worked methodically on his entire lymph system for over an hour. Toward the end of the session, Benjamin's skin color began to look normal. He began coughing, but not the raspy, barking cough that he previously had. The coughing was clearing his lungs. He jumped off the table and began running around. On the drive home, he started fussing as we approached the familiar golden arches. I assured him that we would stop to get his french fries. My mother and I watched in amazement as he consumed an entire large order of fries. When we arrived at his pediatrician's office, he confirmed that Benjamin's lungs were clear. I am sure that he probably wondered why I brought a healthy-looking, active boy with clear lungs into his office that day.

My mother and I were astonished that we had witnessed his healing on the therapist's table!

I was balanced with LEAP therapy for airborne allergens, yeast, and my lifelong allergy to chocolate. My daughter was balanced for her immunizations, airborne allergies, and for red dye 40. She suffered a particularly severe reaction to red dye 40 after eating a red valentine lollipop. She had red, raised hives all over her entire body for almost a week. We are now completely allergy-free!

When Benjamin was five and a half, I had the privilege of attending a lecture on dietary interventions and autism presented by Donna Williams. Donna, who grew up in a suburb of Melbourne, Australia, was diagnosed with autism quite late in her life, at the age of twenty-five. Donna wrote *Nobody Nowhere*, an account of her struggle with the sensory-perceptual and information processing problems common to autistic persons, and has authored seven other books in the field of autism.[24] Donna is also an artist and musician. When Donna began the lecture, I had a very difficult time believing she was the same person whose struggles were detailed in the book. She was funny, articulate, well informed, and seemed extremely comfortable in front of the audience of several hundred people.

She explained that the turning point in her condition was when she was first treated in her twenties using nutritional medicine interventions. She discovered a "dietary disability" was an underlying cause of many of her difficulties, including information processing problems, fluctuating mood states, and an addiction to adrenaline, resulting in a severe anxiety state she calls exposure anxiety. Donna credits a special diet (dairy/gluten-free, sugar free, low salicylate, additive-free) and the use of nutritional supplements with overcoming about half of her difficulties. A low dosage medication addresses most of her remaining difficulties. She had a digestive disorder described as "leaky gut" syndrome, which led her to be diagnosed with secretory IgA deficiency. One of the main functions of secretory IgA is to bind to various food antigens, thus preventing their entry into the general circulation of body.[25]

In addition to her creative work, Donna has worked as a consultant with hundreds of autistic children and their parents helping to resolve dietary and behavioral concerns. She presented some startling statistics. Her research has shown:

- 80 percent of people on the autistic spectrum can't digest dairy and gluten (Shattock, Sunderland University)

- 60 percent of people on the autistic spectrum can't tolerate salicylates (Waring, Birmingham University)

- 20 percent of people on the autistic spectrum have low secretory IgA, with 8 percent having none. (Gupta)

The most fascinating information she presented was how she felt when she ate certain foods. She described how her dependence on and cravings for high salicylate foods created highs and lows that made her feel like a cocaine addict! She listed some high salicylate foods: grapes, raisins, honey, dried apricots, almonds, and strawberries. These were all foods that Benjamin craved. I suddenly had a revelation—for the past month, Benjamin had been eating a fruit and nut bar and drinking a fruit smoothie for breakfast. The smoothie contained mostly fruit and the bar contained dried apricots, almonds, honey, and coconut—all foods that are very high in salicylates! The past month had been really difficult as my husband and I tried to cope with Benjamin's increasingly erratic and uncontrollable behaviors. He would bounce off of the walls by ten o'clock every morning. We couldn't understand what was causing the sudden change in his behavior. I realized that my child was probably high from his inability to tolerate salicylates!

Salicylates are found in varying amounts in many plant foods like fruits, vegetables, nuts, honey, herbs, spices, artificial colorings, flavorings, and preservatives. In natural flavorings, like fruit or mint, the concentration of salicylates can become quite high. The same can be true for some herbal supplements. We experienced the same out of control behaviors when I tried placing Benjamin on some dietary supplements that contained herbs. Although Benjamin is a very picky eater, he often tries to sneak into the bathroom to eat toothpaste, which contains high concentrations of salicylates from mint flavorings.

I immediately placed Benjamin on a low salicylates, food additive-free, dairy-free and gluten-free diet.[26] Within two days, his behavior improved dramatically. Within a week, his impulse control had improved by 80–90 percent. Within one month, he regained the speech abilities that he had previously lost, and he no longer seemed compelled to keep his body moving at all times. He seemed much more calm and content. When he was accidentally given rice cakes that contained corn (gluten), his impulsive and uncontrollable behaviors returned and he lost the ability to speak. After three days he returned back to his greatly improved state.

We've decided to pursue a dietary and biochemical treatment regime by Dr. Edward Danczak, a medical doctor trained in holistic medicine in London, England.[27] The regime is designed to reduce intolerances so that a normal diet may be maintained after treatment. We began supplementing Ben's diet with L-glutamine, a natural amino acid. After thirty days of supplementing with this amino acid, Donna describes having a simultaneous sense of herself and others for the first time. Previously, she would swing between a state of "all self/no other" and a state of "all other/no self."

Donna describes herself as "wild and wooly, with an incredible naughty streak, prone to phobia and compulsion with a great determination to strive for balance and detachment yet a great love of connection and discovery." She does not consider herself "cured" but describes herself as held together with very good sticky tape. She says that those who know her personally would still recognize some of her autism-associated challenges, but these are minor when compared to where she came from. To hear Donna explain the difficulties that people who share this condition face was enlightening. To see her ability to demonstrate many of the wonderful and special characteristics that I see in Benjamin was truly inspirational.

In considering all of the possible treatments for Benjamin, I began to feel overwhelmed by the sheer number of available treatments. I wanted to make sure that I didn't withhold a beneficial treatment or use all of our financial resources on unnecessary treatments. I knew that muscle response testing seemed to be able to predict which treatments would be beneficial to Benjamin, but I was not trained to muscle-test, and it was not feasible to find someone who could muscle-test Benjamin for all the possible treatments and substances he came into contact with on a daily basis.

In my meditations, I began to get the impression that I could ask for help in determining which treatments would be helpful. The "knowings" of my childhood began to emerge. I began by thinking of a therapist or treatment, then asking if the treatment would be helpful. I then sat with the feelings I received, being very careful not to interpret fear as a response. Sometimes I would receive a strong feeling of positive emotions. Other times, I felt nothing. Usually, I would get different feelings for different therapists, even if they were using the same healing modalities. I never went against those feelings in choosing therapies for Benjamin.

Using this method, I had him treated by an esoteric healer and a naturopathic doctor. Even though a trusted friend recommended each of these individuals, I still used my "gut check" method to make a final decision on the treatments. On another occasion, I read that the EMF Balancing Technique had been helpful for autistic children.[28] We were out on a limb financially, but I got very positive responses when holding the treatment in my thoughts. I decided that I would make some inquiries about finding a therapist or a teacher so that I could learn the technique. I decided that if Benjamin needed the treatment, it would work out with ease and grace.

I located a teacher who was scheduled to teach a course a few weeks later in Honolulu when my husband was planning to be there on a short break between business appointments. I had thought about meeting my husband in Honolulu, and coincidentally the class was scheduled to begin on the day after I would have arrived there. I sent an e-mail to the teacher, who was Australian. She happened to be teaching in Europe when my e-mail arrived, and was planning to make a stop in the states to visit a relative. She agreed to stop over in Texas and teach the course and evaluate Benjamin. Benjamin had his treatment within ten days of my first inquiry, and we never even had to leave home. My husband and I have a saying that Benjamin always gets what he needs. We had to believe this after the therapist was in our home to treat him on the day of his official diagnosis, and the Australian therapist appeared within ten days of my inquiry.

I couldn't help but wonder what other important information I had missed while residing "safely" in Western medicine's paradigm. The foundations of the absolutes of my world were being stripped away by a two-year-old healing himself and a six-year-old who could "see" electricity and magnetic fields. As I watched Benjamin repeatedly tune into and evaluate the electromagnetic fields of the body, something that seemed as natural to him as taking the next breath, I found my beliefs being shattered. I was standing on the edge of end-less possibilities. If our bodies could heal themselves, then what else was available to us in the vast universe of our personal experience? What is "truth" when the impossible is realized? This revelation was so huge, so immense that I shuddered at its implications. What other beliefs did I hold as sacred that I needed to examine. Slowly I realized that it was all or nothing.

What do you do when your beliefs are shattered? I did the only thing that seemed to make sense. I became a student of healing, a student of autism, and a student of life. I would carefully crack open the dusty book of the "knowings" of my childhood and look inside. Although I hadn't been able to bring myself to look at it before, now it was different. Like a mother cat hearing the frantic cries of her young, I leapt off into the dark abyss, searching for my son, not knowing that I would find myself.

6 The Conventional Therapies

We shall not cease from exploration and the end of all our exploring shall be to arrive where we started and know the place for the first time.

—*T. S. Eliot*

Upon receiving Benjamin's official diagnosis, we placed him into speech and occupational therapy at a local rehabilitation center. He was being treated simultaneously with conventional and natural medicine therapies. When he was two years and eight months old, testing by the speech therapist indicated that he possessed a severe global speech and language disorder. His prognosis for improving his speech articulation was undetermined upon his admission because he was predominately nonverbal.

Benjamin received combined speech and occupational therapy twice a week, for a 30-minute session. His speech therapy took place in a pediatric gymnasium, with his therapists using Benjamin's inner drive to explore and interact with the environment. The therapists guided him through activities that challenged him to respond to sensory stimuli in an organized way. We were blessed with wonderful, loving, and kind therapists. To assist in developing Benjamin's body awareness, they swung him in a large swing suspended from the ceiling so that he would experience specific movement sensations. To reduce tactile defensiveness, they would rub his arms and legs with different textured brushes. He loved going to his therapy sessions and was very fond of all his therapists. Due to his rapid improvement, he was even selected as the child representative for the rehabilitation center's yearly fund-raising drive.

Several months into his sessions, his therapists recommended that one of Benjamin's weekly sessions be changed to a hippotherapy session at a local stable. Benjamin would receive his therapy while riding on horseback. I was more than a bit skeptical at how successful this session would be. He never showed much affection toward animals, mostly ignoring them altogether. When we arrived at the stable, I was amazed by Benjamin's reaction to the horses. He allowed the therapists to lift him gently onto the back of his therapy horse, Twist. He acted as if he had been riding horseback all his life. He was perfectly comfortable on the horse and, in fact, the therapists allowed the horse to trot at the end of the first session. That day, he developed a close bond with Twist. After his therapy session, he walked over to Twist, placed his hand as high up on the horse's side as he could reach, then buried his head into the horse's side, remaining there for a brief time. A silent communication took place that I could not even begin to understand.

His speech progressed much more rapidly at the hippotherapy sessions. He was asked to give the command to the horse to walk or stop. Soon, he would say "walk it," in response to prompting to tell his horse to "walk on." He was so relaxed on horseback that sometimes he would lie back horizontally on the horse's back and try to fall asleep. There was something about the closeness to the animal and the rhythm of the horse's gait that he found extremely comforting.

When Benjamin turned three years old, he was evaluated by the local school district for a determination of disability and educational needs. He was found to have particular strengths in both his gross and fine motor skills. The district relied on a Preschool Language Scale-3 test that was previously administered for determining his speech and language delay. The test provides language age equivalents in three areas. Auditory comprehension evaluates a child's receptive language skills in the areas of attention, semantics, structure, and integrative thinking skills. Benjamin's scores yielded a language age equivalent of 11 months. Expressive communication addresses the areas of vocal development, social communication, semantics, structure, and integrative thinking skills. His scores yielded a language equivalent of 14 months. The total language results combine the auditory comprehension and expressive communication results to provide an overall assessment of language skills. Benjamin had an overall language age equivalent of 13 months.

Even though he had improved greatly after several months of conventional and various natural medicine therapies, he was still functioning at the upper end of the mild to moderate level on the Childhood Autism Rating Scale. In other words, after almost six months of therapy, he was perched precariously between the most severe moderate level of autism spectrum disorder, just shy of the mildest severe level of the disorder.

Benjamin was placed in the school district's preschool class for autistic children. The class consisted of individualized academic activities, social skills activities, literacy experiences, motor group activities, and language enrichment activities. We were blessed with wonderful and devoted teachers. They all had several things in common: they were respectful and loving, but firm. This combination of love and firmness worked very effectively to form a bridge into Benjamin's world.

Janet Boutton, his lead teacher, and her assistants were lifesavers to me during this time. Whatever problem I was having, Janet would rush to help find the people and resources to resolve it. I began to see her as an angel in human form. Using Benjamin's interests as a guide, she was able to teach him many important skills, including sign language and toilet training. I believe that toilet training is one of the most important skills a special needs child can learn, since it frees the caretaker from the stress of accidents and allows the freedom to venture out with the child. Her method is presented in appendix A.

Sign language was important, because upon Benjamin's admission to school when he was three years old, he was nonverbal. Sign language showed his teachers how quickly he learned and what was important to him. It is difficult for a child to express his needs just by pulling and shoving, and sign language gave him an important bridge into the world of speech. His teachers also used the Picture

Exchange Communication System (PECS), which was developed for communication using pictures and symbols. This system is often used instead of sign language, because sign language requires motor imitation, which can be difficult for autistic children. His teachers created pictures of each item Benjamin might want, such as snacks, and each activity he might want to perform, such as walking or playing with a particular toy. Then they began to use the pictures regularly when working with Benjamin, in order to pair the picture with the item in his mind. Once Benjamin understood that he could communicate with these pictures, he began to use them regularly. His teachers used PECS and sign language simultaneously, since he seemed to show no preference for one over the other.

There are three conventional treatment approaches to autism: drug therapy, psychoanalytical therapy, and behavior therapy. Due to my previous experience with drug therapy, we decided that this method was not necessary or acceptable at this stage of Benjamin's condition. In regard to the psychoanalytical approach, I was not convinced that autism had any emotional component in the traditional sense, since we really didn't know what Benjamin was feeling or how he was handling life situations at that stage. That left only one treatment option: behavior therapy.

Very early on, we were faced with the question of whether to try intensive behavior therapy with Benjamin. On the day of Benjamin's official diagnosis, a friend introduced me to one of her friends who had treated her son with Applied Behavioral Analysis (ABA) therapy. ABA therapy is sometimes also known as Lovaas therapy, after the founder of the approach. Behavioral therapists work with a child using "discrete trials" to eliminate undesirable behaviors and to teach more appropriate skills for living and learning.

I was open to hearing about the successes of the program, but was concerned about the hours of training per week that the child was required to undergo in order to obtain results, anywhere from ten to 40 hours per week. I couldn't fully comprehend sitting Benjamin in front of a hoard of therapists on a rotating basis, forcing him to focus repeatedly on some predetermined item, then be rewarded for appropriate responses. The person who introduced me to the therapy made a tape of her son before using behavioral therapy and actually undergoing the therapy. Before the therapy, the boy's characteristics appeared to be very similar to Benjamin's. I remember thinking that after the therapy, the child looked exactly like the children from my attorney days who had been medicated. Again, I was seeing a wooden-faced child dully complying with instructions, repeated over and over again. There was certainly measurable progress, but at what price?

When I thought about employing behavioral therapy, I just kept feeling like I would be using the therapy out of fear. I would be forcing Benjamin into this rigid protocol with set, predetermined goals so that I could feel better about the progress he was making. It just didn't feel right to use it in Benjamin's case. The only reason I would be using it was to tell myself that I was doing everything possible in order to help Benjamin. I wanted Benjamin to be a boy, to play and have free time like any other child. To the extent it was possible, I didn't want his whole existence to consist of doctors and therapists.

I still have extensive and vivid memories from my childhood. To imagine putting myself at that age into this sort of rigid teaching system resulted in an immediate stomachache. When I was younger, this was my instantaneous truth test. If something felt bad "in my stomach," I knew it was something that I shouldn't do. I knew that I wouldn't want to sit across from someone and be subjected to drills for ten hours a week, much less 40 hours a week, no matter how much it was "for my own good." At some point, I would just have to become numb and try to escape it. I had no desire to use this method to drag Benjamin, kicking and screaming, into my world.

Why should I treat Benjamin differently from how I would want to be treated? Did his condition give me the right to employ such drastic measures in order to make him more "normal"?

I thought about a saying that my mother often reminded me of after Karis was born. "Children are just little people," she would say. "They deserve to be treated with the same respect as any adult would."

That advice was handed down to her from my father's mother, and I never forgot it. Maybe in some people's opinion, it isn't a logical decision not to try everything that would possibly help Benjamin, but it was strictly a decision of the heart, and in my case, of the stomach.

We were fortunate. Before I had much time to contemplate using the treatment, Benjamin showed improvement from his first treatment with LEAP therapy, which made the decision not to use behavioral therapy a very easy one.

I felt even better about my decision upon reading the words of Donna Williams, an adult autistic who survived her own battle for understanding, becoming a college graduate and author:

> Gain the child's trust and tell him or her that you accept who and where he or she is. Through trust he or she may develop interest in "the world," and at first this exploration should be on the only terms he or she knows—his or her own. Only once this is firmly established should you take the safety net away slowly piece by piece. This is the way to make a transition from the child's sense of itself *as* the world to a new sense of itself *in* the world so-called "normal" people share.
>
> This method, in complete contradiction to normal inter-action, is *indirect* in nature. In this way it is less all-consuming, suffocating, and invasive. The child can then reach out, not as a conforming role-playing robot, but as a feeling, albeit extremely shy and evasive, human being. The best approach would be one that would not exchange individuality and free-dom for the parents', teacher's, or counselor's version of respectability and impressiveness.[1]

7 The Gifts

The moment one gives close attention to anything, even a blade
of grass, it becomes a mysterious, awesome, indescribably mag-
nificent world in itself.

—Henry Miller

Many autistic people are savants, possessing "islets of ability,"[1]
advanced skills in a particular area. I have seen the work of Richard
Wawro, a remarkable Scottish artist whose detailed wax oil crayon
works are rich with depth and intense color. He is autistic and has
never had any artistic instruction. Jessy Park paints exquisite archi-
tectural paintings with photographic accuracy. I have read the
poetry of Marshall Ball, a brilliant young man who touches people's lives even though he cannot speak or walk. Although he has
no official diagnosis of his condition, he writes poetry with incredible depth and inspiration. He knows the meanings and spellings
of words to which he has never been exposed. What are these so-
called "disabled" individuals tapping into that most of us are
unaware of?

Benjamin also displays some unusual and unexplainable talents.
His ability to know that my friend's problem involved the area surrounding his left eye was certainly the first of many examples of his

awareness of the body's physical condition. I simply cannot explain this knowledge with conventional thinking.

On one occasion, he was playing in a play area of our local mall. Something caught his attention. From across the room he ran up to a teenage girl and placed his hands on the girl's shoulders. All of his attention was focused on her shoulders. The girl's mother confirmed that her daughter had severe problems with her shoulders.

We can tell by the expression on his face when he seems to be drawn into an area of a person's body. I have found that once I notice that he is paying particular attention to a person's body, if I ask the person about that area of the body, they will always indicate that the area of their body is experiencing difficulty. The focus of his attention is very intense at this time, and it is difficult to redirect him into another activity. He is particularly interested in baby's heads. Once, when visiting a friend's newborn baby who had a particularly difficult birth, Benjamin stared intently at the child, then reached out and tried to grab the baby's head in an unusual fashion, trying to grasp two areas of the baby's head at once. He was attempting to use much more force than I was comfortable with.

On another occasion, at a birthday party, Benjamin noticed a week-old baby that I was holding. He ran across the backyard to where I was seated with his attention focused intently on the baby's head. He reached out his hand and held it above the baby's head, lowering it slowly as I had seen him do before. As his hand approached the baby's head, he began "stimming" as if he were seeing something coming from the baby's skull. I quickly used my training to check the baby's energy field with my hand and felt restrictions on several levels in the location that Benjamin had indicated.

I believe that Benjamin can somehow sense traumas to the body through his perception of the body's energy field. Baby's heads are subjected to trauma during birth, perhaps leaving evidence of this trauma in their energy fields. Benjamin can sense this trauma and sees this trauma as breaks or restrictions in the body's energy field. Donna Eden describes feeling "like a tuning fork." She senses and feels other people's energies as "rhythms and vibrations, frequencies and flows, jolts and currents, colorful swirls and geometric patterns."[2] She describes a colleague who began to smell energies.[3] Could the smell of energy be the reason Benjamin sometimes sniffs objects or people?

Often, I noticed that Benjamin would sniff a favorite food and refuse to eat it. Once I placed grapes that he had refused to eat into a bowl with identical-appearing grapes that he had been eating. As I watched, he picked through the grapes and ate only the grapes that were originally in the bowl, leaving behind the grapes he had previously refused.

A 16-year-old intuitive healer named Adam, in his book *DreamHealer,* describes seeing organized patterns in the auras of healthy persons.[4] He sees broken, disturbed areas in the energy patterns of injured or diseased persons.

I believe that Benjamin experiences the energy of others in a similar fashion.

Once, when Benjamin and I were enjoying a ride on the train, a blind man entered the train and sat directly across from us in a seat facing us. Benjamin immediately got "the look" and moved to the opposite seat right next to the man. He began to lean in front of the man's face and began moving his hands in front of the man's face and neck area. The man sensed his presence, and I immediately moved Benjamin back to the seat beside me, explaining to the man that Benjamin was very sensitive and there was something about him that Benjamin was attracted to. I'm never quite sure how to explain his behavior, even to those who cannot physically see it.

Once, Benjamin tuned into a friend's child who is several weeks older than Benjamin. Although the boys had been playing in the same room, Benjamin had done little to acknowledge the other boy until he noticed something in front of the child's mouth. Benjamin focused on the boy's mouth area as he ran across the room, stopped with his face an inch or two from the child's mouth and began to "stim." Benjamin then reached up and pressed the outside of the child's cheek, directly over the area of his teeth. The boy disliked the close contact and moved away from Benjamin. Acting somewhat distressed and focused on the boy's problem area, Benjamin reached out and tried to hold the affected area of the child's head. I immediately asked Benjamin to stop and explained that the boy did not want to be touched.

The child's mother watched the boys' interaction and asked what Benjamin was seeing. I told her that I believed that he had sensed a break or restriction in her son's energy field around the area of his mouth. She called the boy and had him stand in front of me and asked him to open his mouth. As I looked into his mouth, I saw two very small front teeth. The boy did have problems with his teeth that had puzzled his doctors. His front teeth were ground down to nubs! After consulting with the family dentist, the mother made arrangements for the son to be treated with CranioSacral Therapy.

Benjamin knows that trains are approaching before they can be seen or heard. On many occasions, he has stopped me and refused to cross the train tracks. I now know to stop and wait with him, as a train will approach within a few moments. The first time he demonstrated this behavior, I realized that if he had not stopped me, we would have been directly in the train's path. He would have had no way to hear the train, since we arrived on a train on the opposite track and the departing train would have masked the sound of the second train's arrival. He could not have seen the train, since it arrived from over a small hill. He displays this behavior only when the arrival of the train is imminent. We have noticed the same behavior around cars when he is out walking.

On the morning of September 11, 2001, Benjamin cried when I dropped him off at school and was particularly clingy. He had never done this before. This would have been around the same time as the terrorist strikes in New York City and in our nation's capital. We know that "when emotions are stirred up, earth fields react more potently."[5] Apparently Benjamin wasn't the only one feeling a difference that day.

At Princeton University, the Global Consciousness Project,[6] created by a group of researchers working in the areas of physics and psychology, gathers evidence of the subtle reach of human consciousness in the physical world. They maintain a global network of special instruments designed to produce random data that, under special conditions, are apparently affected by human consciousness. They predict an effect when there is a large-scale coherence and resonance of feeling generated by deep reactions to major news events. On the morning of September 11, the data collectors appeared to reflect the shock and dismay of the nation even before our minds and hearts expressed it.

Maybe thinking that Benjamin could feel this catastrophic event as it was happening wasn't so far-fetched after all. He also awoke crying and inconsolable in the early morning hours on the day of the execution of Timothy McVeigh for the Oklahoma bombing. He wakes up anytime anyone in the family is feeling particularly stressed or out of sorts.

Benjamin has demonstrated knowledge of specific healing techniques. On one occasion, he began to have a severe allergic reaction when he was at his grandmother's house. I watched him carefully on the short drive home, hoping that I would not have to use the epinephrine injector that I carried with me at all times. When we arrived home, he ran into his room and found a small flashlight that shined blue-spectrum light, which I had purchased at the suggestion of a naturopathic doctor for its calming effect. Ben turned on the flashlight, opened his mouth, shoved the flashlight deeply into his mouth, closed his mouth around the flashlight, and held it there for about 30 seconds. Then he opened his mouth, threw the flashlight down, and ran out of the room to play. The allergic reaction had completely subsided.

I had never seen him put the flashlight into his mouth before, and his actions were so deliberate that I sensed while he was doing it that he was trying to get some relief from the symptoms. I later discovered that blue-light energy has been shown to constrict blood vessels and reduce swelling. I was struck by the similarity to the effects of the drug epinephrine, which are to constrict blood vessels, relax the muscles in the airways and lungs, and reverse swelling, virtually the same effects as blue light! How could Benjamin have known this?

On another occasion, Benjamin's grandfather had been hospitalized and had been unable to recover fully from the effects of a recent illness. He had been so ill that he hadn't even felt like seeing Benjamin for quite some time. When he finally did, Benjamin greeted his grandfather at the door. His grandfather scooped him up in his arms. Benjamin began looking at the area around his grandfather's head, reaching out and lowering his hand until he touched the skin on his grandfather's face. He repeated these movements several times. None of us thought much about it, since we had seen Benjamin do this on many occasions, until his grandfather reported later that day that he felt completely healed.

Benjamin has demonstrated that he is able to see under very low light conditions. He has never had a fear of the dark. He has no problem

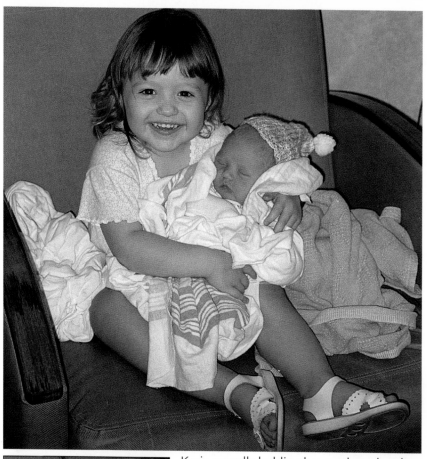

Karis proudly holding her newborn brother.

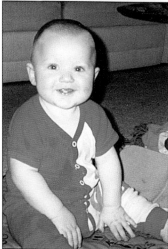

Benjamin at nine months old, having no problem smiling for the camera. Note the eczema on both his cheeks.

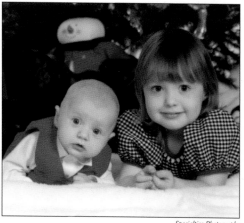

Specialties Photography

Benjamin and Karis in our 1998 Christmas photo. Note his ears, typical of autistic children.

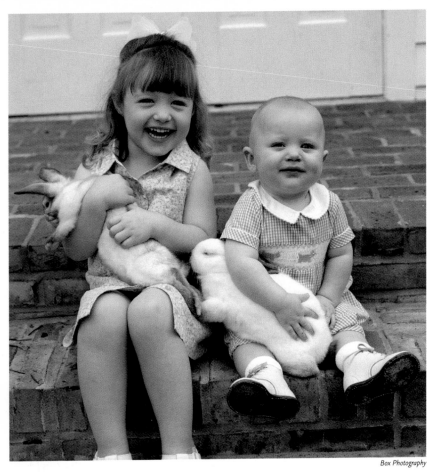

Easter 1999, photo of Karis and Benjamin. At six months old, he loved touching the rabbits and feeling their fur.

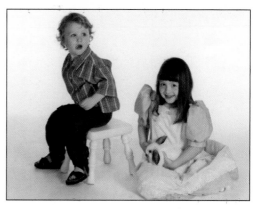

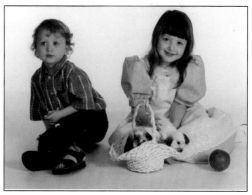

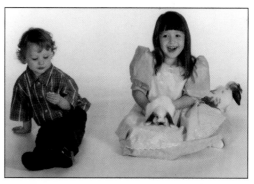

Easter 2001, photos of Karis and Benjamin, taken just weeks before his diagnosis. Despite the photographer's and my best efforts, Benjamin was oblivious to the camera, his sister, the rabbits, and "the world." Only one shot in several rolls of film shows him looking in the general direction of the camera. The photographer could not even get a shot of him fully seated, since he ran all over the studio, as his sister waited patiently for the photographer to get the shot.

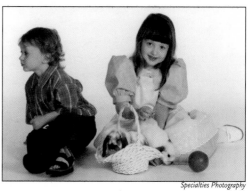

Specialties Photography

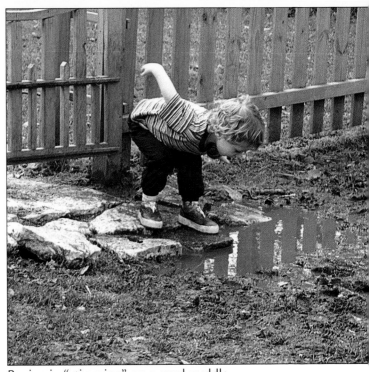

Benjamin "stimming" on a mud puddle.

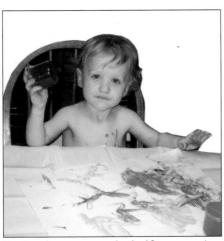

Benjamin at two and a half, attempting to finger paint for the first time. Note the pale skin color and dark circles under his eyes as he stares off into nowhere.

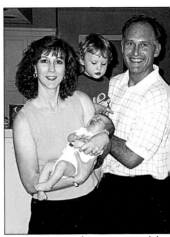

Benjamin at three years old w Mom and Dad. He is tot: focused on the head of friend's newborn baby, ignor the baby's mother who is tak the photo. Note he has slipp his hand between us to touch crying baby's head.

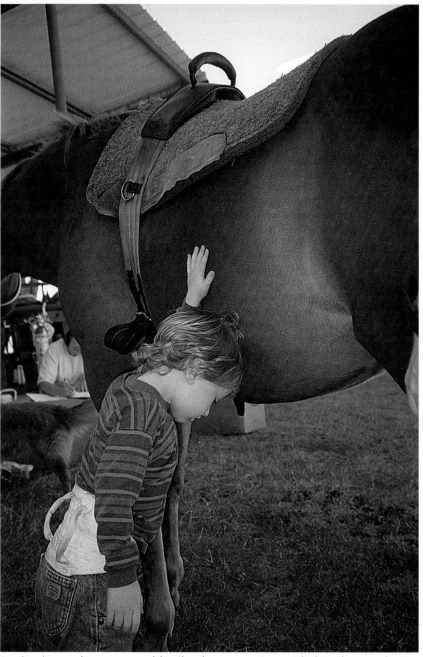
Benjamin at three years old, silently connecting with his therapy horse, Twist, after their first session.

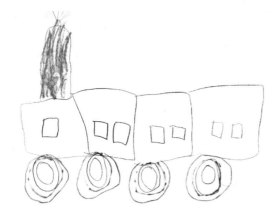

Figure 1. Drawing of an electric train by the author's daughter, Karis.

Figure 2. Drawing by Karis, the author's seven-year-old daughter, of the energy emanating from the author's fingers. Karis has found that the colors of the energy of the left hand are stronger and more intense than the energy of the right hand.

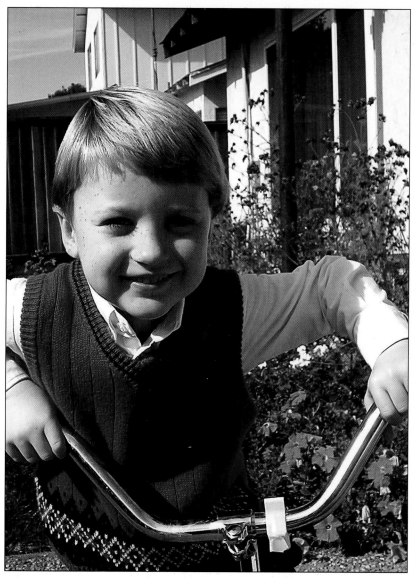

Benjamin at four years old riding his tricycle in California.

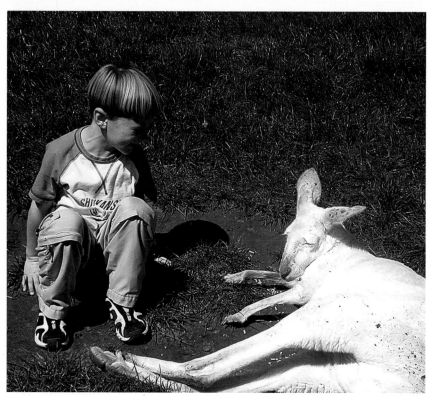
Benjamin at five years old, making friends with an albino kangaroo in South Australia.

going outside at night to play in total darkness, although it makes me nervous. Once when he was at the opposite end in a room of our house, he wouldn't leave the room after repeated requests. I switched off the fluorescent lights, and it became very dark. When I automatically held out my hand to take his, I thought to myself that it was a strange thing to do, since he was probably going to run right into me as I stood in the doorway. I decided not to turn the light on and braced for him hitting me. To my amazement, I felt his small hand reach out and take mine. It was as if it were broad daylight and he reached up to take my hand.

One of our friends with unusual abilities also possesses this ability to see under extremely low light conditions. He relates a story that when he was a young boy, he would go outside in the snow at night to swing on his swing. His family couldn't see him outside, but they would know where he was from the sound of the swing creaking.

We are constantly amazed by the feats that Benjamin is able to perform in the dark. He can locate objects, turn on toys, and negotiate around obstacles in what appears to us to be complete darkness. He seems as content in darkness as he does in the bright morning sunlight.

Benjamin has demonstrated knowledge of things that he could have no way of knowing in a conventional way. A friend gave me a postcard with a reproduction of *The Lamb and the Lion* by Glenda Green. I really liked it and used it as a bookmark. Benjamin walked up to me while I was reading and took the bookmark. He looked intently at it for several seconds. He then pointed to the likeness of Jesus and said "Jesus" very clearly. This was one of the first words he said after beginning his treatments.

Benjamin had never been to church or Sunday school. When he was younger he refused to even stay in a church nursery. One of the few times that I tried to leave him in the church nursery, I heard his cries becoming louder and louder as I sat in church. He had escaped from the nursery attendant and had somehow found me. I can think of no explanation as to how he knew that the picture was of Jesus. The bookmark became one of his favorite items. He would take the bookmark out of my book and carry it all over the house. I often found it in his bed. As I was writing this book, I received a catalog from a bookstore, and it contained this same picture by Glenda

Green. Since I misplaced the postcard over a year ago, Benjamin had not seen this picture in quite some time. I asked him who was in the picture. He quickly replied, "Jesus." He still knew!

One baffling symptom of autism is the fact that these children have to be taught to look at people's faces. From a very young age, Benjamin would look all around my face and body. He would only look into my eyes when he was forced to, when I was holding him. Sometimes, he would still look at the area around my head. Perhaps autistic children don't have a need to look into a person's eyes the way that a "normal" person does. If the eyes are considered to be the windows into the soul, then there is no need to look through a window when the soul is right in front of you. Looking at the energy field of the body provides much more information than simply looking into the eyes could ever reveal.

I have found that Benjamin often looks at the area around my head to determine my mood. After I listen to music, do meditation, or when I am in a particularly good mood, Benjamin will rush over and get into my lap while leaning back to look directly above or beside my head. He gets very excited and hugs me, as if my good emotions and positive state of mind will rub off on him.

Nearly everyone possesses empathy to the emotions and feelings of others. My husband's good humor and playfulness are contagious, and those around him easily sense his mood. We have probably all experienced a meeting with a person who seemed to drain the life out of us. These are instances of psychic empathy. Psychic empaths are not limited by the same boundaries as other people and are so in tune to others that they merge with and feel the physical condition, feelings, and emotions of anyone with whom they come into contact.

Dr. Temple Grandin, an autistic woman who earned a doctorate in animal science, credits this ability to feel and see as an animal does for her successful design of cattle chutes and other equipment that helps alleviate stress on animals while they are being handled and transported.

Benjamin has demonstrated psychic empathy on many occasions.

Benjamin's school was a few blocks from our home. Our usual routine was for Benjamin to throw his leg over his oversized red tricycle with his bright red and black backpack slung over his shoulders and pedal at breakneck speed to his school. Often he would pedal so fast that one foot would fly off the pedal, with the other foot dutifully riding the other pedal until its momentum slowed enough for him to slap his errant foot back on it to continue its frenzied pace. One day he was pedaling at his usual pace when he suddenly stopped. He began to fuss, and he got off his tricycle. He started crying loudly, and I recognized the pitch of the cry as one he used when he was physically hurt.

Confused by his behavior, I asked him what was wrong. He continued crying and tried to lead me back in the direction of the house. I put him back on his tricycle, but he refused to move, crying hysterically. I was totally baffled by his behavior. I picked him up and held him for a few minutes, wondering what I was going to do with the tricycle if I had to carry him the rest of the way to school. For the next few minutes, no matter what I tried, he refused to move forward and insisted on going in the opposite direction. Finally, I put him on the tricycle and began pushing it from behind. He finally calmed down by the time we reached his classroom. When I returned home, I discovered that his sister had severely injured her toe about five minutes after we left the house, which was precisely the time that he began crying. Benjamin was experiencing the pain and fear of his sister's injury.

We already knew that he was very tuned in to his sister's feelings and emotions. We often joked that Karis would need psychotherapy when she got older because we were always asking her please to try not to cry because it would set Benjamin off, and we'd have crying in full stereo sound. The problem was that Benjamin usually continued crying long after Karis had stopped. Her slightest whimper could send him into a crying frenzy. We noticed that he did not demonstrate this with everyone else. If he heard another child crying, he would stop what he was doing and seem to "tune in" to the other child. This would happen even if he could not physically see the other child. After tuning in, he would either ignore the child, or burst into tears. I believe that he was able to merge with the child and determine whether there was physical pain, fear, or simply a ploy to get attention. The younger the child was, the more likely Benjamin was to cry.

One summer day, we decided to go with some friends to Muir Woods, outside of San Francisco. Benjamin loved the redwood trees, and we thought he would enjoy getting out and walking in the forest. About 20 minutes into the drive, Benjamin began to sob hysterically. I stopped the car and sat on the sidewalk as he stood beside me. He threw his little body over my shoulder and continued sobbing. Nothing I did seemed to make any difference. I kept asking him if he needed anything, but he just kept crying. Finally, I put him back into the car and drove back home. I was totally baffled by his behavior until I received a call later that day telling us that his grandfather had been diagnosed with a double aneurysm. He received the news at precisely the time that Benjamin became so upset. He had merged with his grandparents and felt their confusion and fear over his grandfather's physical condition.

When he was three years old, we were returning from the two-hour drive from his therapist's office. We had been driving quite a while when Benjamin began fussing and crying, and acting extremely distressed. About a half-mile farther down the road we came across the scene of a very bad accident. Benjamin continued fussing, and I noticed that he seemed to turn his head deliberately away from the accident scene as we passed. I believe he was sensing the fear and pain of those involved, and possibly the feelings of those working the accident scene. After we passed by, he became calm and remained that way for the rest of the trip.

I had experienced this phenomenon myself. As I was driving down the expressway one day, I saw the back of a man walking in the center median between the two lanes of traffic. He was a road maintenance worker. I immediately began to feel excruciating, stinging pain in both of my arms from the elbows down. As I passed by, out of the corner of my eye, I saw the man holding both arms up in front of his body. I believe that he had suffered some sort of injury; perhaps particularly vicious Texas fire ants stung him. As soon as I became aware that the pain I was feeling was his, the pain vanished.

Benjamin has always had a fascination with electronics. As soon as he was able to pull himself up to a standing position, he was able to operate the VCR. He could put the tape in, fast forward to the scene he wanted to watch and rewind to repeat a scene. Once, at a new therapist's office, he made one running pass by a stereo system. When he ran past the second time, he reached out and touched the one button that would turn the system on.

Even when Benjamin was very unaware of the world, he loved art. When he was first diagnosed, he had speech and occupational therapy sessions at a rehabilitation center. Before his sessions, he would run up and down a long hallway at the center. He would look upward as he was running along, as if he were running under a huge canopy. I noticed that there were framed pictures of artwork positioned high up on both sides of the hallway walls. Children treated at the center created the artwork. I wondered what he was seeing while looking upward and running. Although he often ran looking sideways, I hadn't noticed him running and looking upward except in this particular hallway at the center.

I began to catch Benjamin examining certain prints and original art. He would climb up near the art, then look underneath it, as if something were extended out three-dimensionally from the flat surface. He would take his face and move it around a few inches from the surface of the art, as if he were feeling something with his face, rather than seeing the art with his eyes. I noticed that he regularly displayed this behavior when looking at prints of famous art or art created by children.

While we were visiting a local bookstore, Benjamin grabbed a book off a shelf. It was titled *Willy the Dreamer*, by Anthony Browne. He had never looked at a book before. He opened the book and began looking at the pictures, many of which were inspired by great works of art, including Salvador Dali's *The Persistence of Memory*, and René Magritte's *Le Chateau des Pyrénées*. The book's main character is Willy, a charming chimpanzee who traverses these great paintings with ease, accompanied by his ever-present bananas. Benjamin has expanded his book preferences to include other books now, but this one is still a favorite.

I began to realize that Benjamin had to be seeing something extending out three-dimensionally from certain pieces of art. I thought that he was probably seeing something like different colored rays of sunshine emanating out from the art. In one of my meditations, I asked for information about what it was like to be Benjamin.

I got more than I ever bargained for. The scenario could best be described as a "day in the life" video of Benjamin's daily life experiences. Attorneys, particularly personal injury attorneys, sometimes make a video of an individual who has been injured by someone else's negligent act, in order to show a judge or jury what living a day in that person's life would be like. I felt the shock course through Benjamin's body at the intensity of the first spray of water from his daily shower hitting his sensitive skin. The sharp, penetrating sting of the spray on his skin felt more like penetrating porcupine needles than water spray, and was incredibly painful. Even the altered state of awareness I was in couldn't quell the overwhelming feelings of guilt at all the times I simply lost my patience when he would wince and cry out when the spray of water hit his skin. I'm so sorry, Ben, I'm so sorry. I had no idea what it felt like to you.

Suddenly, I tasted the juicy lemons that Benjamin loved to lick, but they tasted almost sweet. How can that be? Candy tasted almost salty. No wonder he hardly ever finishes a piece of candy, I thought. I experienced the bitter, unpleasant taste of the food he refused to eat and enjoyed the intense, pleasurable sensations produced by his favorite foods. The salty popcorn that he loves produced a simultaneously salty and sweet sensation.

I became Benjamin when he is in the presence of someone who is experiencing a strong emotion. I felt a very unpleasant stretching, pulling, and tugging in the area surrounding my heart. He was experiencing not only what we understand as an emotional reaction, but a physical reaction to the emotion as well. One purpose of his life was to learn compassion, I recalled from that early morning meditation before he was born. That sensation would certainly serve to make one compassionate, I thought.

I understood that his delicate and hypersensitive state was the reason why medications had such an undesirable effect on his comfort level and behavior.

Then I found myself standing at one end of a room. A work of art hung halfway up the opposite wall. What I experienced took my breath away. Rays of light didn't extend out from the art as I had guessed, but blocks of red, blue, and yellow translucent colors extended out three-dimensionally from this piece of artwork. These blocks were similar to big, thick, fabric-colored blocks that children stack one on top of the other, except they ranged from very translucent blocks of color to almost opaque blocks of color. Each block extended out three-dimensionally in differing depths from a few inches to many feet from the wall. Golden light streaks projected from the blocks of color along with smaller lavender- and magenta-colored corkscrews and triangles that seemed to penetrate the blocks. These geometric shapes were immersed in the blocks of color, yet somehow stood apart from them.

I knew that somehow I was sensing the energy and the emotion that the artist had attempted to capture two-dimensionally on the canvas, just as Benjamin did when he looked at a piece of art. The experience was emotional, overwhelming, and amazing, unlike anything I had ever experienced in my life. I wanted to run through the colors and feel them. Only after this vision faded did I realize that I had failed to see what artwork had produced this canopy of color. I was an adult, trained in observation and in facts, and I didn't even notice what piece of art was hanging on the wall. Just like Benjamin, I had failed to see the tree for the forest. Now I know why it is so difficult for him to focus on our stale, bland world, I thought. There is so much for him to get through before he even gets to what we see.

One day as I was driving my daughter to school, she began talking about the light she was seeing emanating from her arm. I asked her the color of the light, and she said purple. I told her that some people are able to see things that other people can't, and that I believed that Benjamin was also able to see these things. I explained that Mommy and Daddy weren't able to see them, but we believed that there were people like her and Benjamin who could.

"You know how he gets all excited when he sees water swirling down the drain of the bathtub?" I asked. "I think he's seeing something that we don't see."

"I know why he gets all excited and twists his arms when he looks at the orange tree in the backyard," she said.

"Why?" I asked.

"He sees all the little points of light that are in the tree."

"You see the light, too?"

"Yes, there are little tiny bits of light that shine out from the tree, and that's why he gets excited when he looks at it."

"What color is the light?"

"All different colors," she replied.

"Can you see light coming out from any other trees?" I asked.

"Yes," she said, "but some trees have more than others. The big tree in our school yard has lots of light coming from it, but mostly from where the kids have scraped the bark away."

"Were you able to see lights coming from the trees in Texas?" I asked, trying to hold back the urge to begin a complete cross-examination.

"No," she replied.

"Have you been able to see light coming from the trees ever since we moved to California a few months ago?"

"Yes, and the light coming up from the ground."

"What light coming up from the ground?"

"The pink light that I see coming up from the ground by our family room door."

When we arrived at her school, she unbuckled her seat belt. Leaning forward to give me a hug and a kiss, she said, "I can see light coming from right here, too," pointing to a spot on my chest. "It's yellow and purple and green."

"We'll talk about this again, soon," I said, as she slammed the door shut.

Wow, first electricity and now trees and people, I thought, as she turned and waved, then disappeared behind the weathered gray door.

I thought about the time in Texas when our family cat had been bitten on the paw by another cat. He was limping and the bite appeared to be forming an abscess. I had planned to attend a Lymph Drainage therapy class the next day, which was Saturday, but arranged to have my husband take the cat to the veterinarian, since I knew that animal bites could be serious. When I arrived home, he had misunderstood my instructions and now the veterinarian clinic was closed. I worried about how the paw would look after another few days without antibiotics.

I called Karis into the room and asked her to help me send healing energy to the cat's paw. We sat there for several minutes, concentrating our thoughts on healing the paw. I wasn't really sure that healing would occur, but Karis must have been sure. The next day I woke up and looked outside to see the cat jump up onto a bench outside. The cat was no longer limping! I called Karis and we brought the cat inside to inspect his leg. There was a faint outline of the bite, but the abscess was gone and the leg appeared to have healed. We had quite a party that morning. Karis used this same healing energy on the feral cats that lived around our new California home.

We realized that Karis seemed to have an extraordinary gift for healing, especially if Benjamin became ill and his illness could possibly keep us from doing some fun activity. With her assistance and Lymph Drainage therapy, Benjamin was rarely sick for more than one day, and healed completely without the use of antibiotics.

I am not providing details of my children's seemingly unique abilities for sensationalistic reasons. In fact, I believe that everyone has the potential for doing these types of things. My purpose is to suggest a different way of treating children, and educating children. I believe that children who are considered autistic are square pegs that we are attempting to force into round holes. In doing this, we may just be chipping away the most important parts of their being. Perhaps they are here to help us realize that we've gotten away from what is important.

8 The Influences

> Of all the communities available to us there is not one I would want to devote myself to, except for the society of the true searchers, which has very few living members at any time.
>
> —*Albert Einstein*

The therapist who initially treated Benjamin with LEAP therapy called me shortly after one of his treatments. While in a hypnagogic state, that brief period of time between resting and being asleep, he had received a strong impression that something in the physical environment where we lived was not beneficial for Benjamin. His impression was that it had something to do with the land.

I experienced many of my "knowings" while in that state. In fact, when Benjamin was an infant, I repeatedly experienced a dramatic vision. The image of a locomotive, moving swiftly and closing in rapidly, appeared to me many times during a one-week period. As we lived in an area where we routinely had to cross railroad tracks, I was emotionally shaken by the vision. I even purchased an infant's car seat that would be easier and quicker to remove from my vehicle in the event I was faced with that situation. Within a week, a friend's parents and children were struck by a train while riding in a car. His parents were killed, but his children survived. Thankfully, the visions stopped, but I wished that I had been able to perceive more information, such as who was threatened by the train, so that I could have warned them and experienced less anxiety myself.

Upon hearing the therapist's concern about our physical environment, I immediately contacted one of my friends who had helped me to understand some of Benjamin's more unusual tendencies. He made periodic trips to our area of the country, so I knew he would be familiar with the land. I asked him about the physical environment in the area of Texas where we were living. He confirmed that the area where we lived tended to be stressful on the body. He said that the negative effects tended to be less severe out in the rural areas to the south of town. His impression was that because water and gas reserves are taken from the ground in great quantities where we lived, the earth has to replenish that displaced energy by using any other available energy sources. People could be an available source. The phenomenon of negative earth energies and their impact on the human body is known as geopathic stress.

He mentioned that positive and negative ions might also have an effect on the body. Negative ions, which have a positive effect on the body, are present near the ocean and mountains. The area where we lived contained more positive ions, with its flat terrain and lack of water source. Positive ions are less beneficial for the body. Although most people can feel a slight difference when in these differing conditions, for someone as sensitive as Benjamin, my friend believed that the effects could be much more dramatic.

I was aware that this friend could feel subtle energy that was undetectable by virtually anyone else. One day as I was talking to him on his cell phone, he warned me that we might soon lose our connection, which we did. When he called back a few moments later, I asked him how he knew that we were about to be disconnected. He said that he can feel the cell phone energy waves, and when he feels them weaken to a particular level, he has learned that he will lose his cellular signal.

I contacted my other friend who could perceive subtle energy, and he came to our home to get an impression of the conditions there. When I initially contacted him, he was not concerned that there could be any negative effects on Benjamin. He had lived in the Houston area for more than 20 years and was vocal in his opposition to our moving from the area. When I answered the door, he gave me some surprising news. On the drive into town he had discerned such negative effects that he had already decided that it would be best if we moved from the area. He mentioned that the area south of town had a better energetic feel than the rest of the area.

None of the three men who provided information about the land or geopathic stress in our area knew each other, yet they all had concerns about the effects of our physical location on Benjamin's body. Two of the men even agreed that a particular rural area south of town had a better energetic feel.

What was all this subtle energy stuff that these men were feeling? I knew that I felt much better physically when I was someplace other than where we lived, but I thought it was just my love of travel and the excitement of being somewhere different. Again, I turned to Dr. Hunt's research in *Infinite Mind* to search for a scientific basis for these impressions. Dr. Hunt had discovered that "electromagnetic environments in which we live powerfully affect our biological fields"[1] and can have different effects on the quality and size of the human energy field. The Santa Ana winds in southern California contain strong positive ions, causing the human field to become small. After many days of these winds, she reports that people became irritable and sometimes ill. Sending a person with a small field to swim in a pool, take a cold shower, or walk barefooted in the grass increases the field and improves the person's mood, probably due to increased negative ions. Negative ions present in the mountains or near the sea also serve to expand the energy field. This helps to explain why atmospheric changes can disturb many sensitives. When positive ions in the atmosphere replace the negative ions in the human aura, the human field is weakened and becomes ungrounded.[2]

Well, it seemed there was a scientific basis for what these men were telling me. I hadn't even considered the atmospheric changes. The area where we lived was known for rapidly changing weather and thunderstorms.

We were willing to do anything that would help Benjamin, including moving across the country, so we put our home on the market and began doing research on where to point the compass in search of our new life. We narrowed the search to somewhere with nice weather, since Benjamin liked to spend so much time outdoors.

The job market had to be large enough that my husband could find a job, there had to be a therapist with LEAP training in the area, a good public school system for Benjamin's next year of preschool, and it would have to be near a type of private school that we had selected for Karis. As she had endured so much change since Benjamin's birth, we knew it was time to make a positive change on her behalf. There was one area that met all of our criteria, and that was the San Francisco Bay Area. I made reservations to take a flight out within two weeks to visit Karis's prospective school.

As the airplane made the final approach into the San Jose airport and the tops of the trees peeked from behind the clouds, I had a strong impression that the move was the right thing to do. I spent a few days in a hotel situated beneath giant stands of redwood trees and returned home feeling renewed and recharged.

Our move was completed within a few months. We expected that Benjamin would need some time to adjust to the new environment. We were wrong. The day we arrived, we began unpacking boxes and organizing the household. I walked to a neighborhood restaurant to get sandwiches. As we sat on the front porch eating our dinner, Benjamin walked up and stared at the sandwiches. He reached out to grab the sandwich and took a big bite. Then he did the same thing to my husband's sandwich. It was the first time Benjamin had ever eaten a sandwich.

His sleeping patterns improved greatly. He slept all night long almost every single night. If he did awaken during the night, he would awaken without the screaming and crying that was so common when we lived in Texas. He began to be interested in any food that we were eating. Pizza became his favorite food. He was willing to try almost any food that was given to him, with the exception of meat. During one of our trips on the light rail into downtown San Jose, Karis spotted an ice cream vendor. I pulled a dollar bill out of my purse and exchanged it for an ice cream cone. As Karis began eating it, Benjamin walked up to her, took the ice cream cone away from her and began eating it. We watched in disbelief as he devoured the entire ice cream cone. He had never shown any interest in ice cream, and I certainly hadn't given him any because of his previous milk allergy.

Could it be possible that just moving to another area of the country with more negative ions, thereby increasing the strength of

Benjamin's electromagnetic field, resulted in such a dramatic difference in his overall general health and well-being? I knew the improvement was real, but why did it occur?

Dr. Hunt tells of a woman who was suffering from cardiac dysrhythmia for several months and could not be stabilized with medication.[3] In a cross-plot analysis comparison of two different simultaneous recordings, the dysrhythmic heart showed the same anti-coherent field pattern as her anti-coherent energy field. A healthy heart and a healthy energy field are both coherent. By improving her field coherency, the anti-coherency in her breathing and heart came under automatic control, allowing her to heal without the scheduled pacemaker operation.

By far the most amazing effect of the move was that Benjamin began talking. His use of spoken language increased dramatically from the moment we arrived in California. He began speaking in sentences within a few weeks of our move. One day, he started to fuss. I asked him what he wanted, and he looked up and me and said, "I want to go ride the train now." Karis and I were ecstatic, dropped everything, and headed to the train station. All the information from the past four years was sitting in his little mind, but until there was less weighing on him, he had no energy to get it out. How frustrating his life must have been before he was able to use his expressive language. Apparently, there was no problem with his receptive language skills. He had been understanding everything that was said to him, but wasn't able to respond. No wonder he threw temper tantrums!

He began naming everything he saw. The interesting thing about Benjamin's progress in California is that I deliberately did not resume treatments when we moved here. He has not had any speech, occupational, CranioSacral, or LEAP therapy since our move, except for the minimal services he received through the school district as part of his preschool curriculum and some basic Lymph Drainage techniques that I use when he is ill. He was doing so well that I wanted to observe whether the improvement would continue without any further intervention, and it has.

Maybe there's a reason for California being known as the land of the "way out there" people. Apparently, something about the geography and conditions here allows one to feel and "see" differently. Karis was able to perceive subtle energy in the electromagnetic field of people and trees after our move to California. She was unable to perceive these same energies when we returned to Texas for visits. Perhaps the answer lies in the ions.

9 The Possible Explanations

What know ye of my soul's unending strife which lies untried in
   thine?
How can ye with a knowledge of thy life write out a creed for
   mine?
         —carved in wood in grotto of Nevada canyon (author unknown)

The learned authorities on autism could only offer high proba-
bilities of mental retardation and a 50/50 chance that Benjamin
would eventually have to be institutionalized. Just like his life-
threatening milk allergy condition, I was told just to wait and hope.
I'm not much good at waiting. I knew that it was up to me to find out
what was happening. I knew that I could not deny the things that I
was seeing my son do. I knew that it was extremely unlikely that the
synchronicities that I was experiencing with Benjamin could occur by
chance. I believed that there must be some guiding force at work, and
I knew that our unusual abilities held the key.

Imagine that a blank white wall stands before you in a dark room.
A flashlight is switched on and shined on the wall, and a stark white
circle appears in the darkness. The white circle is the reality in which
you live at that moment. The rest of the wall appears nonexistent. The
light moves slightly. Awareness shifts and a new reality exists.

In her book *Spiritual Awakenings,* Barbara Harris Whitfield explains how each side of the brain functions differently:

> The human brain is divided into two separate hemi-spheres, the left and right, and joined in the center by a large nerve track called the corpus callosum. Both sides of the brain have different but complementary functions. They process information differently and in varying levels of intensity. Each side thinks in its own way. *Each side also speaks to us differently.*[1]

Dr. Leonard Shlain explains the functioning of each hemisphere of the brain:

> The right hemisphere integrates feelings, recognizes images, and appreciates music. It contributes a field-awareness to consciousness, synthesizing multiple converging determinants so that the mind can grasp the senses' input *all-at-once.*
>
> The right brain, more than the left, expresses *being*—that complex meshing of competing emotions that constitutes our existential state at any given moment. . . .
>
> The right brain more often than the left generates feeling-states, such as love, humor, or aesthetic appreciation, which are *non-logical.* They defy the rules of conventional reasoning.
>
> A feature of nonverbal communication is that no sym-bolization interferes with the direct appreciation of reality. The right brain perceives the world *concretely.* For example, a facial expression is "read" without any attempt to translate it into words.[2]

The right-brain perception of the world is all-at-once. Benjamin has demonstrated on many occasions that he perceives in this fash-ion. Even Albert Einstein was known to think in images, rather than in words. Dr. Shlain maintains that:

> The right hemisphere is also the portal leading to the world of the invisible. It is the realm of altered states of con-sciousness where faith and mystery rule over logic. There is

compelling evidence that dreaming occurs primarily in the right brain. . . .

Another major right-brain feature is its ability to appreciate music; the perception of sounds, which the right lobe integrates into an all-at-once harmonious feeling state.[3]

Right-brain abilities seemed responsible for Benjamin's profound appreciation of music, his ability for extremely authentic, strong feeling-states, and his appreciation of art.

Barbara Harris Whitfield explains how the functioning of the right hemisphere may be impeded:

The soft gentle voice of intuition is activated through the right hemisphere of our brain. Our logical left hemisphere doesn't want to believe in intuition . . . spiritual awakenings, cyclic time or creativity. These come from the right hemisphere, and the left feels threatened, wanting to remain in control . . . We in the West have been taught to suppress our right hemisphere traits, cutting ourselves off from half of who we are . . . when we awaken . . . we open to both sides of the brain . . . Our right hemisphere can delight us with new ways to absorb knowledge and intuit reality.[4]

She relates that upon having a spiritual awakening, her brain began to function differently.[5] Her time perception changed or slowed down. Time didn't feel linear, but seemed to exist in cycles. Even little things seemed spectacular. Creativity flowed. I have experienced all of the same phenomena since my experience shortly before Benjamin's birth. Is it possible that my experience occurred with perfect timing, creating a pathway through my rigid left-brain dominated mind, enabling me to understand what I was seeing in Benjamin?

What if some children are born with particularly sensitive systems, perhaps even genetic or physiological differences, then their delicate systems are systematically shut down by a bombardment of toxins, as a result of immunizations or other environmental poisons? If Benjamin cannot take a dose of a common, widely used antibiotic without suffering ill effects, then I cannot even imagine how his body must have reacted to a cocktail of chemicals just hours after his birth. What if the damage results in the shutting down of portions of the left hemisphere of the brain, the portions that are crucial to perceiving the world in a "normal" fashion? What if this damage leaves these children with virtually one hemisphere of the brain functioning, the right hemisphere? Could this explain the unusual abilities that I was witnessing? Could it be that Benjamin's abilities and my knowings were simply right-brain phenomenon that are not widely accepted or understood in our left-brain dominated society?

Dr. Margaret Bauman, a pediatric neurologist at Harvard Medical School, has found an interesting difference in a portion of the brains of autistic persons. She examined postmortem tissue from the brains of nearly 30 autistic individuals who died between the ages of five and 74. She found densely packed neurons in the amygdala that are smaller than in normal persons. Dr. Bauman maintains that the subtle differences do not appear to be brain damage.

The amygdalas "look unusually immature," comments University of Chicago psychiatrist Dr. Edwin Cook, "as if waiting for a signal to grow up."[6]

John J. Falone, in his book *The Genius Frequency,* attributes the ability to move into and out of different levels of awareness to the same amygdala complex. He believes that the amygdala's purpose has been usurped in the average person's brain to expand sensory data, at the expense of the ability to access higher levels of conscious awareness. If an autistic person's amygdala appears immature, has it somehow bypassed a more normal sensory function and instead provided a pathway to these higher levels of conscious awareness?

Donna Williams was labeled retarded, disturbed, and insane before her diagnosis of autism at age 25. In her book *Nobody Nowhere,* she describes her ability to "know" things, without any of the usual cognitive clues.

I would have daydreams in which I was watching children I knew. I would see them doing the most trivial of things: peeling potatoes over the sink, getting themselves a peanut butter sandwich before going to bed. Such daydreams were like films in which I'd see a sequence of everyday events that really didn't relate in any way to myself. I began to test the truth of these daydreams, approaching the friends I'd seen in them and asking them to give me a step-by-step detailed picture of what they were doing at the time I had the daydream.

Amazingly, to the finest detail, I would find I had been right. This was nothing I had controlled, it simply came into my head, but it frightened me.[7]

At a friend's home, she "saw" the image of the friend's grandfather waving at her, describing his size, build, stance, looks, and dress to her friend who could not see the image.[8] He died three days later. She also experienced a precognitive dream in which she shared a house with a man, knowing "his name, his family background, the sort of person he was, and his way of life" several years before actually meeting him.[9]

In researching why Benjamin might be able to "see" auras and to see under extremely low light situations, I discovered from Shlain's book that in the human eye, there are two functionally different types of cells: the rods and the cones.

[T]he contrasting functions of the rods and the cones correspond to the division of tasks between the right and left brain.

Rods, named for their cylindrical shape, are extremely light sensitive. Like trip wires, they detect the slightest movement in a visual field. Distributed throughout the periphery of each retina, they see in dim light and appreciate the totality of the visual field, seeing images as gestalts. Rods share with the right brain the ability to perceive reality *all-at-once.*

The eye divides every scene into two major elements: figure and ground. Figure is visualized sharply and in detail; ground provides the context within which the figure resides; the cones best see figure; the rods best visualize ground.

Because rods supply the big picture, they are the key component of a visual, physical, and mental state known as *contemplation.* The rods enlist the entire individual to help them perform. Muscle tension diminishes. The brow becomes unfurrowed. The pupil dilates. The skeletal muscles of the eyes relax, unfocusing vision. These actions serve to let maximum light into the eye. In this right-hemispheric mode, the individual is better able to see the entire visual field rather than any one detail. Looking at nothing, the eye in this state sees everything. This receptivity affects the whole body. Consciousness idles and a person slides into the integrated mental state of *being*.[10]

This was interesting information, since I was aware that when attempting to see an aura, or energy field around the body, a person is instructed to relax the mind and the eyes, focus on the ground rather than the figure, and use the peripheral vision, instructions that would allow the use of the rods of the eyes. Perhaps the reason autistic people have no need to look into a person's eyes is that they are using the rods of their eyes to take in the entire visual field at once, rather than using the cones to focus in on a person's eyes!

Temple Grandin, an autistic adult, maintains that the sense of sight in autistic children is so keen that they can actually see the flicker of the 60-cycle electricity in fluorescent lights.

What exactly is happening when Benjamin gets emotional when Karis does, or he feels the pain that she is experiencing, even though he is physically several blocks away? How can he see the energy fields of the body and promote healing? How can any of this be possible, I asked myself.

Again, I turned to Dr. Hunt's research to find out more about the other type of electromagnetic energy she discovered in her lab at UCLA. At eight to ten times faster than other biological electricity sampled from the body, this extremely high biological frequency (EHF) was found in experiments dealing with mind phenomena and human consciousness. This small signal would have been undetectable until the development of telemetry.

Dr. Hunt states that at the extreme ends of the consciousness continuum there are "two foci of reality."[11] At one end is a grounded state in material reality (350 to 600 cycles per second) and at the other end an altered state (up to 200,000 cycles per second), where there is nonmaterial awareness apart from earthly time-space. In an altered state, "experiences seem to exist in any time, now, then, forever and whenever."[12] The higher states, without a solid grounding in the body may be referred to as "out of body" states. "Expanded consciousness encompasses a complete spectrum of vibrations with grounding in the lower frequencies combined with great power in the higher ones. Here any level of reality one desires is available."[13]

Donna Williams describes her existence "like an out-of-body experience" in which she had "lost sight of the controls that could bring me back down to earth,"[14] and explains that she was the way she was because of a "constantly changing state of awareness."[15]

Tito Mukhopadhyay, a 14-year-old autistic boy, hardly knew he had a body at all.[16] He relates that when he was younger, only hunger, the feeling of the wetness of the shower, or constant movement allowed him to sense that he possessed a body. He felt that he existed because he could move. Without movement his senses became so disconnected that he would lose his body, so he would flap his hands or rotate his arms to calm himself.

Before undergoing various therapies, Benjamin certainly didn't appear to have much awareness of material reality and was totally unaware of any concept of time. From all outward appearances, his brain seemed to be fairly low functioning during this time. We couldn't even determine whether he was mentally retarded. Because Benjamin's body betrayed him and couldn't provide him with the usual input from his left brain, could he have been knocked "out of body" by the assault on his system, forcing him to operate on some other nonmaterial level of consciousness, allowing him to "see" stressed areas of the body?

This could explain why he was so low functioning, yet knew things that were impossible for him to know. Is this similar to the phenomenon experienced by persons who suddenly lose hearing or sight? Do other abilities become more acute to help compensate for the loss? In Benjamin's case, his entire body was so stressed that bodily senses were of little help. Did his functioning right brain provide a pathway to his higher mind? Does this explain the "islets of ability" demonstrated by many autistics? The "islets" exist in drawing, music, calendar calculation, rote memory, drawing ability, perfect pitch, the ability to play an instrument that one has never been taught, and the ability to play a complex piece after hearing it only once. These are examples of "knowing" without any left-brain instruction, yet they are very real and their existence cannot be refuted.

Many experts agree that there is nothing in the brain that accounts for experiences and capabilities of the mind, such as intuition, insight, knowing, creativity, or imagination. In fact, the mind has often been described as a separate entity that hovers just outside the brain.

Dr. Hunt asserts that there is no neurophysiological research that conclusively shows that the higher levels of mind are located in the brain tissue. "Although some levels of awareness occur in the brain, higher levels of consciousness have not been found there. To the contrary, some philosophers surmised that consciousness is on a continuum from material to nonmaterial reality in which the mind is always involved, sensing nonmaterial happenings primarily, while the brain taps the material ones."[17]

Like Dr. Hunt, I was intrigued that we could have a consciousness that monitors our awareness outside physical reality. Could this be the source of Benjamin's knowledge of things he had never been taught or explain the "knowings" of my childhood? If this were the case, then the operation of the mind would mirror the world of physics.

Einstein stated that the only reality is that of energy organized into fields. If all matter were disintegrated, we would be left with a field, the primary source.

Dr. Hunt wondered if it were possible that the "long undetectable energy of the human mind springs from the electron energy of the body's atoms?"[18]

> Energy in this form, permeating all tissues, does not need to be conducted through the nervous system. The mind-field would then be a literal super-conductor. If the electron spin-off from the body atoms is the source of the mind's energy, then the mind might also reabsorb free electrons from the universe. Since there are no mechanical losses in such a system, the mind energy is literally recycled in the environment.
>
> We already know that the mind is capable of energizing and communicating with matter, including the brain, the body, and other material things. Electromagnetic waves from the universe and those from the atomic structure of the body in field form could meet these requirements. At some level,

all material boundaries are permeable. Electromagnetic energy in the form of waves constitutes information circuits which can penetrate physical boundaries and, like "worm holes," flow through and back into the environment. These qualities of an energy field also describe the mind, that is, the mind is beyond material substances yet interactive with them in an open system.[19]

Did Benjamin somehow perceive this mind energy, these free electrons, spun off from the body atoms?

[W]e discovered that when a person's field reached higher vibrational states, he no longer experienced material things such as bodies and ego states, or the physical world. He experienced knowing, higher information, transcendental ideas, insight about ultimate sources of reality, and creativity in its pure form.

All of these experiences we attribute to the higher mind because they are not available through the ordinary senses at lower field vibrational levels. In fact, the consistently highest vibrations were recorded from people who were accepted "seers" and "knowers," people . . . [who] know things about us and the world without the usual sensory clues.[20]

Dr. Hunt then asked how it was possible to read another's intangible mind-thoughts unless these were expressed in some form. She concluded that a person must be decoding our mind field with his, resulting in a "direct mind or field communication,"[21] rather than reading information stored in the brain.

Benjamin has demonstrated this capability. One day the three of us were riding in the car after picking up Karis from school. As we sat quietly in the car, I recognized Benjamin's voice as he began repeating in a loud, halting voice, "Ryan . . . DeeAnna . . . Ryan . . . DeeAnna."

"Mom, why is Benjamin yelling out what I was thinking?" Karis asked.

"Were you just thinking about Ryan and Deanna?" I asked.

"Yes, and now he's saying it," she said, with a hint of irritation creeping into her voice.

Ryan and Deanna were two children who attended Karis's school. Benjamin didn't know them and didn't know who they were. We didn't even know that he was able to say their names.

How can he possibly know what she is thinking or how I am feeling before I even have a chance to outwardly react, I wondered. I turned to Dr. Hunt's *Infinite Mind* for a possible explanation:

> At the deepest level, all things are composed of vibrations organized into fields that permeate the entire structure. Fields, whether biological or otherwise, have their own integrity. They are organized, not random, and they have the capacity to selectively react, interact, and transact—to respond passively, and to cooperatively unite with other fields. In other words, the mind aspect of the field, the aspect with the highest vibrations, dynamically guides all choices and transactions as it influences and is influenced by all other fields.
>
> Emotion provides a force which flows and fluxes; it captains a field organization to maintain its integrity. Whether the mind-field can continue without becoming disorganized is determined by the strength of the emotion.
>
> Patterns of the mind dictate complex human behaviors; brain patterns activate simpler ones. Every experience has concomitant emotions, and every emotion temporarily restructures the field. Activated emotions increase the electromagnetic flow of the field. Likewise, emotions arise from an altered electromagnetic environment.[22]

Apparently, Benjamin was able to feel when these vibrational fields were changing, causing him to react. He was reacting to emotions because they actually reorganize the field. He was somehow merging with a person's field, and if the person's field became disorganized by strong emotion, so did Benjamin's. The difference is that most people have learned either how to shut themselves off from the fields of others, or to reorganize their field once they become emotional. Benjamin does not possess this ability. This could explain why he continues to be upset long after the person who originally felt the emotion has returned to normal.

Could this phenomenon also be responsible for Benjamin's aversion to large groups of people? Large crowds of people emit "scattered, yet concentrated, energy fields" that may be debilitating because we "respond so immediately to human field happenings"; being in large groups can "push us past the dynamic edge of chaos into a disintegrating anti-coherent field."[23] It certainly seems disintegrating and anti-coherent as I watch my child melt into a puddle at my feet when we find ourselves in a crowd.

John Falone, in *The Genius Frequency,* maintains that the aura is a shell that results from the meeting of electromagnetic attraction, thermodynamic radiation, and high frequency light radiation. It exists in a fourth-dimensional zone of equalization where any substance or thought form received or transmitted must interact with this barrier. He maintains that the brain stores only codified past experiences, while the auric field encompasses the fourth-dimensional mind, which has the ability to operate in past, present, or future dimensions. Therefore true genius is a frequency of the mind and resides outside the physical brain. Similar to a computer, the auric field is a portal of multidimensional awareness capable of processing universal data, but it must have an access code to admit this information into a person's consciousness. Could a slight variation in the structure of the amygdala in the brain or the mental state of contemplation provide this access code?

Most of us operate entirely in an intellectual capacity, using only our brains, filled to capacity with traces of past memory, in order to make sense of our world. Falone provides the following example:

> [A]n intellectual entity will stroll through the garden labeling, rather than apprehending, the reality of the moment. In lieu of the experience of the flower, the intellectual views it by suspending most of the *feelings of connection* . . . as the intellect asserts itself: "Lo, it is a flower—spelled f.l.o.w.e.r.—named rose of the genus *Rosa,* having thorny stems and producing variously colored petals, composed of . . . etc., etc. . . .[24]

Someone who experiences while in a state of contemplation instantly bypasses the intellect as their awareness registers the overwhelming awe of nature's creative majesty. This person identifies with the rose by merging with the energy field of the rose and *becoming* it. Benjamin experiences nature in this way. I longed to experience the essence of a tree to the extent that he was able to experience it. I often found him behind trees, hugging them. Scooping him up, I'd ask him what he was doing. He would lean over to the tree, look at it, hug it, then reply, "I love you, tree," with such depth of emotion that it would bring tears to my eyes. To Benjamin, the essence of the tree is every bit as real and alive as I am. In a world where all living things are as important as people, there is no need to put people first. There is no concept of first or last, best or worst. Everything is just experienced, without judgment or classification.

Donna Williams contends that her emotional hypersensitivity arose "from the inconsistency of changes in consciousness," leaving her and other autistic children to function "on a far more sensory and subconscious level for their waking lives as well as their sleeping ones." She points out that her "constantly changing sense of time and space" and tendency for having night terrors indicates that "some of this emotional insecurity arises from drifting in and out of a dream state."[25] Could dramatic shifts from one level of consciousness to another be causing the discomfort and disorientation common to autistic people?

What about Benjamin's perceptions while "stimming"? When Benjamin perceives intense energy, such as the energy in the waves, the spin of metal against metal on train tracks or the energy systems present in the body, he perceives this movement and it translates into physical excitement in his body.

Why do many autistic persons flap their hands while "stimming"? The hands have several important meridians that end or begin in the fingers. These meridians affect the heart, small intestine, large intestine, circulation, and lungs. In Chinese medicine, the meridians are the channels, or pathways, that transport vital energy throughout the body. Moving the hands in a flapping or twisting fashion may serve to pump up the meridians and ramp up the energy to achieve a higher dimensional communication with the object. The movement may be an attempt to match the high vibrational frequency and "become" the thing he is observing, similar to a form of communication.

Others have indicated that the arms and legs of the human body serve as the pathway for outside frequencies to enter the body and are known to absorb the greatest amount of energy from the environment. Specifically, the frequencies enter through the left hand and exit out the right hand. If a sensitive person were able to sense this movement of energy, it would explain the excessive movement of the hands and the overwhelming need to run that many children experience, as well as the intensity with which these children "stim."

Imagine a world where everyone sees in black and white. Then a child is born with an ability to perceive color. The child spends hours studying, looking at, and being fascinated by the various shades of color that he sees all around him in his environment. Everyone would think that this child was a bit "soft in the head" for paying so much attention to something that no one else could perceive. There must be something wrong with him, since everyone knows that the hues of the world are dull and lifeless. For his own good, he must be taught not to pay attention to the colors. He must be taught to act as if there is no color in the world. He must agree with us that colors don't exist because this is our belief. It is much too distressing for us to consider that he may be seeing something that we cannot.

When Benjamin perceives swirling water, he sees sparks of energy in the water, but his main attraction to it is a pulsing in the energy of water. He can sense and feel it.

How unlikely is this explanation? Dr. Masaru Emoto, a researcher in Japan, began studying water by taking photographs of frozen crystals of water collected in a variety of situations. He believed that if he froze water and took a picture of the crystals that formed, he could obtain information about the water. He and his team have taken and stored over ten thousand photographs of water crystals. In his fascinating book, *Messages from Water,* he compiled photographs of distilled water crystals, both before and after they were exposed to various stimuli. His photographs show that when water is exposed to beautiful music, by such composers as Mozart, Beethoven, and Bach, it is transformed from a nondescript crystal into a beautiful, intricate, more symmetrical crystal pattern, with each sample having its own unique formations.

Further, he found the same phenomenon when exposing the water to various words, both in English and in Japanese. Words such as "you fool" and "you make me sick, I will kill you" and "dirty" produced water with poor or no crystallization patterns. The patterns created were aesthetically ugly and appeared damaged. Words such as "beautiful" or "love/appreciation" produced beautiful crystals that were similar to the water that had been exposed to classical music.

The most interesting photographs were of tap water in Shinagawa, Tokyo, both before and after five hundred people throughout Japan offered "chi and soul" to the water at the same moment on February 2, 1997. The water was transformed from a polluted sample with virtually no crystallization pattern into a beautiful, symmetrical, six-sided crystal. Dr. Emoto believes that the subtle energy in the water is related to consciousness.

I wondered if this is what Benjamin sees in the water. How does this affect all of us, considering the fact that our bodies are comprised of over 70 percent water. Could it be that our thoughts and feelings are instantaneously affecting all of us at this most fundamental level?

10 The Change in Me

Children should be seen, and heard, and believed.
                              —*bumper sticker seen in Santa Clara, California*

I've spent the majority of my life doing what was expected of me. I was told what would keep me safe, how I should live, and how I should think. By controlling everything within the parameters of what I already knew, I believed that I would be safe. I only colored inside the lines. I lived in fear of what was outside the lines. I have found that the good, juicy parts of life are in the unexpected, outside the lines. When one isn't challenged by a life-changing event, whether it is a special needs child, a health challenge, or the death of a loved one, it's just oh-so-comfortable to stay where you are. In the past, it's taken an earth-shattering event to slow me down enough to become conscious of the life that I'm living.

My conscious questioning began when my mother-in-law died from cancer, less than a year after my husband and I were married. I began then wondering what life was really all about. Two good jobs, advanced degrees, the big house, and the "successful" lifestyle somehow felt very shallow and empty, not to mention the worrying about what everyone else thought about my actions. The need for acceptance and approval was exhausting. I somehow knew that my "living inside the lines" was not where I needed to be.

Benjamin's entry into our lives forced me to begin the searching process in earnest. I wouldn't have done it for myself, but I had to do it for him. His "illness" was the best catalyst for change. We had to stop listening to what we *should* do because it just didn't work; not only didn't it work, but it failed miserably. I had no way of knowing that the search would take us into dangerous territory, where a small crack formed in the dam of our belief system. Once the water started to trickle through, nothing could stop it. It became a raging torrent, taking out all the beliefs that stood steadfastly before it.

Most people think that they are nothing without their beliefs—their beliefs in conventional medicine or alternative medicine, religious beliefs, beliefs that controlling one's environment will make one feel safe, belief in having no other choice. I have discovered that without my beliefs, I am free to be anything and do everything. One's beliefs are just as limiting as one's fears. They're both just boxes that one puts oneself in. Even my beliefs about autism are subject to change because they are simply beliefs. They do not define who I am.

After we received Benjamin's diagnosis, I virtually dropped off the radar. I no longer did the things that I did before. The priorities that I had before his diagnosis were completely rearranged. Most of my friends lamented the losses that I experienced when Benjamin's condition was diagnosed. In some respects, I lost my freedom. I could no longer be a part-time mom. The part-time work situation that was so perfect after my daughter was born was totally unworkable for Benjamin. I needed to be a full-time-and-a-half mom. My whole world consisted of my children. The one who required all my time, and the other who demanded so little of me. Sometimes, I did feel a loss, a loss of certainty, a loss of normalcy. Many times, I felt anger.

I realized that my anger resulted from my loss of freedom and the demands placed upon me. Eating out as a family at a restaurant was virtually impossible during the early days of his diagnosis. Other than when Ben was first diagnosed, the only time that I have cried was out of frustration at not being able to meet some old friends in a restaurant. He refused to go into the restaurant. When I carried him in, he began screaming. I still do not know what caused his reaction that day.

At times, I was angry at the judgments of others. I was angry that they assumed that Benjamin should be pitied. They failed to see the joy in his eyes or his capability for unconditional love. They failed to see how precious he was, but how could they really be expected to see past their beliefs? Once again, I found that I must accept *what is* and let go of my belief that anyone should understand what it felt like to have a child like Benjamin.

Many well-intentioned people had opinions about what we should do about Benjamin. I have found that I need to look carefully at the life of any person who wants to offer me advice. If that person is living the kind of life I want to live, then I listen to the advice. If they are not, then I know that although the person probably has the best of intentions, that person probably has no better understanding of the situation than I do and may be operating out of fear. I've made enough decisions out of fear to know what one feels like and how counterproductive it can be.

At times, I was angry at the financial implications of having a child like Benjamin. Not only did I lose the freedom and challenge of my career, but we instantly cut our family income in half. A large portion of the therapies that worked successfully on Benjamin was not covered by insurance. We did what we felt would help Benjamin, as we watched our bills mount. I knew that I needed to be with him, yet I felt the pressure of our finances. When we moved from Texas, we sold our home, leaving us virtually debt-free, but penniless. Was it worth it? Absolutely. The situation proved to us that our possessions were only that—possessions. A big house and new cars don't bring happiness, especially when you come home to a child who is uncomfortable in his own body, and who makes sure that you know it. I knew that if I could understand Benjamin's condition, then the rest would take care of itself.

More importantly, the situation was a catalyst for change in me as a person. Each morning I woke up asking what I could do to discover something about my son. Then I would ask what I needed to discover about myself. Daily, I received answers. Some things that I discovered about myself weren't so attractive, but the lessons I learned helped me to grow so that I could handle the next challenge. These past few years have been a very valuable graduate lesson in life, even though I had sworn to my friends that I was through with my education!

If I continued to resist Benjamin's condition and try to fit him into what everyone else wanted him to be, we would be continuing to replay the same scenario we were in several years ago. I would have no understanding of his condition, and I would be striving to have a child that I did not have, working to mold him into something that he is not. We would be living in the same place, doing the same things, living the same life until we were dead and buried. Doing that is worse than a physical death. It is continuing to live by just going through the motions.

One of the most difficult things for me to learn has been that sometimes I need to get off my own agenda and just "be." In the past, I was so rushed and busy that I never noticed nature. I was in survival mode, not in living mode. Now, I enjoy watching Benjamin squat down on our neighbor's sidewalk to inspect one rock in a group of a hundred rocks. I've become aware that he always plays with the same rock. He holds the rock as if it is a valuable, precious gemstone, sometimes holding it briefly to his face. I now know that he is seeing or feeling the essence of that rock. If I forced him to hurry up and quit messing around, I would have totally missed the fact that he makes a distinction between different rocks and trees. There are certain trees that he always greets upon arriving at the park, just as there are certain rocks that he must touch as he passes. I've learned much from this boy.

11 The Status Quo

Perfect love casteth out fear.

—*1 John 4:18*

In the early days of Benjamin's diagnosis, my doctor asked me how I was handling the diagnosis. I began explaining that we were doing just fine, and that we believed that everything happened for a reason, including Benjamin's condition. The doctor, who delivered Benjamin and is a good friend, then asked, "How do you handle the bitterness?"

How do you answer that there is none? Bitterness is not something that is a part of my life. There is a time when I would have allowed the *poor me* thinking to set in, but this would mean that I was a victim in life, rocking along, taking whatever hand chance chose to deal to me. My life is my responsibility, and my happiness is my responsibility. I am not the victim of random acts of good or bad that are somehow bestowed upon me purely by chance. How I handle the situations that occur are up to me.

Shortly after our move to California, I began looking for a pediatrician for Benjamin. I searched alternative medicine sources and found a pediatrician who advertised that she also practiced alternative medicine. I called her office, requesting an appointment to discuss

Benjamin. The receptionist, upon hearing that Benjamin was autistic, put me on hold. The pediatrician picked up the line and began backpedaling.

"How old is your son?" she asked.

"He was four in August," I replied.

"What is his diagnosis?"

"PDD-NOS."

"You have used alternative therapies with him?" she asked.

"Yes, he has been treated with CranioSacral Therapy. Are you familiar with it?"

"No, I don't really use alternative therapies, just some old home remedies," she responded, "and I really don't know much about autism either, just that it is a very disappointing illness."

"That really hasn't been our experience," I countered. "My son has made tremendous strides in the past year and a half."

"Well, if you get into a situation where he needs something specific, then call me."

Fat chance, I thought to myself. She didn't want to contaminate herself by being associated with a "hopeless" case.

This wasn't the first time we had sensed a misunderstanding about Benjamin's condition. Before his official diagnosis, he was denied life insurance coverage because his medical file indicated that he suffered from a speech delay. What a speech delay has to do with life expectancy, I can't imagine.

The thought occurred to me that caregivers of autistic children are in a much better position to observe their children than medical professionals are. When an autistic child is taken in for treatment, whether it is for speech therapy or a doctor's appointment, it is always accompanied by the stress of the child having to adapt to a new, unfamiliar environment. Usually waiting rooms are crowded and bustling with people, so these professionals never get to see the same child that we do. Especially in the situation of treating a child's acute illness, this is not a routine task. It is a progression of events that is totally unfamiliar to the child and does not carry any predictability, and it entails something that the child is least good at—waiting.

No wonder medical professionals believe the situation is hopeless. They see these children at their worst, which I admit can seem pretty bad as the events are unfolding. They don't get to observe the child as he snuggles with his daddy at night, reading and laughing and acting just like any other child. We are the ones who are best able to observe behaviors and subtle differences and interact with the child in all situations. The professionals are looking for "cures" for the behavioral aspects of the condition, which doesn't necessarily emphasize the overall well-being of the child.

In selecting schools for Benjamin, I believe that it is much more important that he be in a loving environment with caring teachers than in any particular curriculum or teaching method. Benjamin performs best for people that respect and care about him, just as we all do.

The interesting thing about autistic children is that most teachers agree that traditional schooling simply doesn't work for these children. Benjamin's classes are very child-directed and use his interests to facilitate learning.

Donna Williams, an autistic adult who earned a college degree, states about her attempts to be educated:

> [I]f I concentrated too hard, nothing would really sink in. Unless the task was something I had chosen, I would drift off, no matter how hard I tried to be alert. Anything I tried to learn, unless it was something I sought and taught myself, closed me out and became hard to comprehend, just like any other intrusion from "the world."[1]

Donna Williams's favorite teacher "brought in records and asked us to tell him what we thought the music and songs were saying to us. What I liked, most of all, was that there were no wrong answers. Everything was supposed to be only whatever it was to each child. [He] never emphasized ability, but instead allowed me to show him what I was capable of . . ."[2]

Using a child's interests to facilitate learning stands in sharp contrast to traditional schooling where subjects are determined in advance, dissected into individual subjects, and presented by a teacher to be received (or not!) by the student. The purpose of this method of schooling was to educate the masses to be workers in a postindustrial society. Many of the fears associated with having an autistic child is that they will not become productive members of society unless they can attend traditional schools.

I would like to go out on a limb and say that I believe that it is much more important to raise a sensitive child with his or her natural talents and abilities intact than it is to produce another factory worker, another doctor, or another lawyer. The knowledge level of our society is increasing at an exponential rate. How do we even go about determining what subjects are important to learn? When I think about my own education, with the exception of reading, writing, and simple arithmetic, I cannot think of any situations where I actually used the subjects that I was taught in school. The same situation occurs in higher education. I learned very little about the practice of law in law school. I did learn logical reasoning and a little procedure, but not what it is like to meet with a client, prepare a case, and argue it before a court. Ask any lawyer and I think they will agree. The degree was simply a means to an end. It was not about obtaining knowledge, it was about passing exams.

Why should we be concerned that our sensitive children can't pass traditional exams? What if they become artists or healers or visionaries? Isn't this just as important? This concept was so aptly articulated by John Taylor Gatto, a former New York State Teacher of the Year in a speech to the Vermont Homeschoolers Conference:

> To get better schools that actually served us instead of suffocating us, we would need to successfully challenge certain scholastic and corporate assumptions. We would need to abandon, entirely, the idea that any such reality as mass-man actually exists. We would have to believe what fingerprints and intuition tell us—that no two people are alike, that nobody can be accurately described by numbers, that trying to do this sets up a future chain of griefs. We would have to accept that there is no such thing as a science of pedagogy, nor is one possible—that each individual has a private destiny. We would need to transfer faith to such principles and behave as if it were true. We would have to come to our senses and admit that knowledge is not a substitute for wisdom. We would have to believe each American has the right

to live as he or she deems wise providing only they do no harm to others.[3]

Perhaps autistic children are here to demand what Mr. Gatto suggests: that we find a better way of educating our children.

12 The Synchronicities

The Healed Mind Does Not Plan

—*A Course in Miracles*

Carl Jung, a Swiss psychiatrist, and Wolfgang Pauli, a physicist, collaborated to develop their concept of synchronicity in a marriage between the approaches of physics and psychology. Jung originally defined synchronicity as "the coincidence in time of two or more causally unrelated events which have the same or similar meaning"[1] and a "meaningful coincidence."[2] Synchronicities reveal, in particularly dramatic ways, links between inner mental patterns and events in the external world. These involve quite different orders of connection than those associated with our familiar notions of causality, since synchronistic events cannot be explained by any conventional account of causal relationship.

In his essay "Synchronicity: Bridge Between Matter and Mind," F. David Peat asserts:

> Despite our appeal to a "scientific view of nature," such events do occur, and while it is true that any one of them can be dismissed as "coincidence" such an explanation makes little sense to the person who has experienced such a

113

synchronicity. Indeed the whole point of such happenings is that they are meaningful, and play a significant role in a person's life. Synchronicities are the jokers in nature's pack of cards for they refuse to play by the rules and offer a hint that, in our quest for certainty about the universe, we may have ignored some vital clues. Synchronicities challenge us to build a bridge with one foundation derived into the objectivity of hard science and the other into the subjectivity of personal values.[3]

He continues his inquiry in his essay "Synchronicity: The Speculum of Inscape and Landscape," by stating:

On the one hand we have the inner world of our direct experiences, of dreams and aspirations, memories and visions; the world of love and loss, of poetry, art, music and of spirituality. And, on the other, the world of matter and energy, the domain of physics and chemistry, the world of black holes, galaxies, elementary particles and quantum fields. And so, in speaking of Synchronicity, one asks if a bridge is possible between these worlds, between mind and body, between matter and spirit.[4]

He questions whether there is an inherent fragmentation in our thinking, if there are simply two sides to one reality or two modes of experience, rather than two different worlds. He points to a "sense of pattern and meaning which dissolves the boundaries between inner and outer and transcends our normal orders of space, time, and causality."[5]

He explains further that synchronicities are often associated with periods of transformation, as if the internal restructuring produces external resonance or a "burst of energy"[6] that extends outward into the physical world.

During the entire experience of Benjamin's birth, discovery of his condition, and healing of his physical discomfort, I was struck by the number of synchronicities that seemed to guide and shape our handling of each situation. The fact that I began meditation classes the month that he was conceived, allowing us to establish a direct channel of nonverbal communication was the first synchronistic event. The fact that I experienced a spontaneous spiritual awakening shortly before Benjamin's birth was the second. The third was the woman in the health food store who led us to a CranioSacral therapist for his milk allergy.

The seemingly miraculous healing that Benjamin experienced paved the way for the fourth synchronicity, the therapist who was present in our home when Benjamin was diagnosed, leading to the first major breakthrough in his autistic symptoms through the use of LEAP therapy. This sequence of events then led to the appearance of the Australian EMF Balancing Technique therapist who appeared in our home within ten days of my discovery of the therapy, a miraculous synchronicity by any standards. Other synchronicities were meeting the two men at exactly the right moment to help me understand Benjamin's more unusual abilities and seemingly irrational fears, and my two dear physicist friends who were literally sitting right across from me, to help me make sense of the physics of the situation.

Our decision to move to California was also bolstered by the same invisible guiding force. While in Texas, I had been attempting to find a part-time job with the flexibility to allow me to be with Benjamin when he wasn't in school. I found this to be fairly difficult when practicing law. I had known of a part-time appointed judge position that was being created, yet for some reason, the job simply could not get approval, even though it appeared that everything was in place. I was very fond of all my coworkers at the courthouse from my assistant district attorney days, and I felt that the job would be one that I would greatly enjoy. I waited for many months, thinking that the job would be approved. Once my husband and I made the decision to move to California, the position was approved the next day, a process that took almost an entire year! I love reminding my husband that we were less than 24 hours away from not making the move to California, because if the position had opened before our decision was made and I had been hired for the position, it would have been very difficult to leave the security of that job.

The next amazing synchronicity involved where we would live once we arrived in California. During my visit there to investigate possible schools for my daughter, I looked for housing. I began to get fairly overwhelmed, by both the number of possibilities as to where to live, and by the seemingly outrageous price of housing. I decided that if the move were meant to be, then the perfect housing would be presented to me. I enumerated eight criteria for the perfect house, then let it go. The house must have a fenced yard, both front and back, so that the children could play, and I wouldn't have to worry about Benjamin escaping into the neighborhood, as he often did in Texas. The house must be within walking distance of the light rail line, and within a short driving distance to Karis's school, have at least three bedrooms, in addition to a separate office, be within walking distance to Benjamin's school, be offered at a price that we could afford, have a nice, modern kitchen, and windows across the entire back of the house, so that I could check on Benjamin while he played outside.

I forgot about it for a few weeks, never allowing myself to worry about our housing in California, even when it slipped casually into my awareness. A few weeks later, I received an excited phone call from my mother. She had written her only friend in the Silicon Valley area, telling her that we were planning to move there. Upon receiving her letter, that friend called my mother, explaining that her best friends were moving to Arizona, and their home would be available. I knew we had found our house. We made flight reservations to visit California to see our new home. The home met all eight criteria. As an added bonus, the house had virtually the same floor plan as our present home, except that the positions of the dining room and kitchen were swapped, resulting in my being able to watch Benjamin in the backyard while I was in the kitchen, a great improvement over my current home.

Benjamin's exceptional teachers made our decision to leave Texas a difficult one, but somehow I knew that there would be wonderful, loving teachers waiting for Benjamin in California, and there were. We enrolled Benjamin in a California public preschool class for children with various learning or physical disabilities. His classmates had various special needs, but weren't autistic.

The next synchronicity was an introduction to Frank DeMarco, my publisher, who provided great encouragement to write this book. I was attending a course when my dear friend Ron Bryan tracked me down in another part of the building so that I could meet Frank. By the time our conversation ended, I was in the enviable position of having a publisher willing to consider publishing this book before the first page was written.

The next wonderful synchronicity was that upon moving to California, Karis developed the ability to "see" subtle energy forms, allowing her to give me more insight into some of Benjamin's more unique abilities.

The last synchronicity was our move to Australia, which resulted in the opportunity to meet Donna Williams, who lives in Australia, and to learn of her success in overcoming her autistic symptoms through dietary interventions. Convincing me that a particular diet could make such a drastic difference in Benjamin's behavior would have been extremely difficult without meeting Donna and hearing her describe how certain foods made her feel when she ate them.

I can certainly relate to the words of Barbara Harris Whitfield because I, too, am having a "wonderful love affair with a breeze that I can't see or prove but that has impeccable timing and is certainly wiser than I."[7]

13 The Boy Today

It is never too late to be what you might have been.

—*George Eliot*

We no longer seek normalcy for Benjamin. We seek comfort. I'm no longer afraid to glance at Karis, treading water gracefully as we go along. I no longer fear that if I dare to look at her to see how she is doing, I will look back to find that Benjamin has slipped beneath the surface of the water. I know there is nothing to fear.

I am no longer afraid to look into the eyes of strangers and see pity. I pity them that they can't see what I have learned to see. They don't see or understand what their gaze falls upon. They see a child who at first glance seems absolutely perfect by the world's standards. Then, without warning, he seems anything but perfect.

As we boarded the train one day, Benjamin ran to the section of the train where the bicycle riders hang their bicycles for the short trip. Across from the racks are five seats. Benjamin sat next to a man who was sitting in three of the seats with his bicycle beside him. Benjamin wanted to look out of the window, which was centered over the middle seat. He was leaning very close to the man. Another bicycle rider got on the train. He was having great difficulty lifting his bicycle into the rack. I got up to help him lift and center the bicycle on the hook. The first man stood up to move to another section of the train, and as he did, Benjamin moved over into half of his seat. As the man who just boarded sat down, he tried to put his backpack into the seat that Benjamin was partially blocking, but Benjamin refused to move. I tried to move him over out of that seat, and he began to yell. The man continued to shove his backpack where Benjamin was seated.

"Stubborn," the man commented.

"He's autistic. If I try to move him, he'll continue to scream and be upset until we reach our stop," I replied.

"Well, maybe it's partly that and stubborn," the man countered.

"Are you familiar with autism?" I asked.

The man stared blankly at me, shaking his head.

"Autistic people don't have a good understanding of where everyone else is, and what they should do to be courteous," I continued.

"He probably just isn't used to riding the train," the man snorted, still trying to stuff his backpack where Benjamin was seated.

Benjamin was really showing someone their own stubbornness, I thought, as the grown man and a four-year-old remained engaged in their battle of the wills. The train was almost empty, yet the man wanted the same seat that Benjamin wanted.

"He rides it everyday, but today he decided that he wanted to sit here," I said. "We usually sit up there," I added, pointing to the elevated section of the adjoining car.

He probably knew someone needed a lesson on stubbornness, I thought to myself. We continued along on the train, Benjamin and the man's backpack remaining pressed against each other in the narrow seat.

These days, Benjamin is able to wait in line until we can order his favorite french fries. With my encouragement and explanations, he can withhold the impulse to cry. He can hold back his sense of urgency and the emotions that he feels long enough to accomplish a task. He is starting to understand his relationship to time. Occasionally, we go to a restaurant, just the two of us. I explain to him exactly what is happening as the events unfold.

"See, Benjamin, first the man brings us our water. Then he'll take our order," I tell him.

"Ice cream," he says.

"First eat lunch, then have ice cream," I explain.

Benjamin begins to fuss.

"Must have good behavior to get ice cream," I continue.

"I caaaan't," he whines.

"Yes, you can, Benjamin. I know you can have good behavior so you can get ice cream."

"I'll try," he says, in his most pitiful voice.

"Good trying," I reply after a few minutes of his remaining in control.

We order and share a wonderful black bean and corn quesadilla. We celebrate with ice cream. Recently, we celebrated a successful outing at a restaurant. He remained in his chair and had good behavior for an entire hour, as we sat enjoying each other's company.

Within three months of our move to California, we got the best present a parent could receive. Some friends were visiting from Japan. Benjamin had never met them before. When they arrived, Benjamin made eye contact and sat between them. He began singing "Itsy Bitsy Spider," complete with hand movements. He interacted with the couple and delighted in their response. He then completed the concert with a finale of "Twinkle, Twinkle, Little Star." We were absolutely amazed. He sought out the interaction with the couple, who were strangers to him. He performed for them and was aware of their responses. We were ecstatic.

On his fourth birthday, he watched with great excitement as his birthday cake was brought to the table. He sat down in front of the cake. He grinned broadly as we began singing "Happy Birthday," waiting patiently for the end of the song. He watched each face as we sang to him, until the conclusion of the song. When the singing stopped, he took a deep breath, and blew out the candles. Giggling with glee, he delighted in the attention, taking it all in, then devoured the birthday cake, a carrot cake with cream cheese frosting, specially prepared by his grandma. I couldn't help but think about the stark contrast between this birthday celebration and the one two years before.

One day, Benjamin and I went to a local park that has a tall concrete slide, built into the side of an embankment. Children love climbing the large concrete steps to discover the slide, just over the top of the hill. The surface of the slide is rough concrete. Benjamin slid down the slide on the seat of his khaki pants, making for quite a bumpy ride. I watched him make several trips down the slide in this fashion. Then, to my amazement, I looked up to see him standing at the top of the slide with a piece of cardboard in his hands. He had watched the older children sliding effortlessly down the slide on the pieces of cardboard and decided to try it himself. When he reached the top, he carefully placed the piece of cardboard on the slide, sat down on it, and careened down the slide. He had learned by watching others, something autistic children aren't supposed to be able to do!

I remembered the words in one of Benjamin's reports, "Although Benjamin might be able to participate in some incidental learning, the consultant would recommend against thinking that Benjamin is going to learn any type of toy play skill or social skill in a purely incidental manner." So much for that recommendation, I thought.

On another occasion, a kind woman who helped me with the feral cats at our new home came by to help me set a trap in order to capture a particularly clever female who had eluded me. Benjamin had never met this woman before. As Benjamin watched her taking the trapped cat outside to her car, he began to get extremely upset. I explained that she was helping me with the cat and that I would bring the cat back after we took her to the veterinarian.

He looked at the woman and said, "Hug you." Before she left, he hugged her and gave her a kiss. He knew that she was helping us with our furry friends. He made the connection and responded in an appropriate fashion.

I loved watching him hold the tiny kittens that we rescued and nursed back to health. I loved watching the complete and total trust that they have in him. He has taken on the responsibility to feed these cats. He seems to know when they are hungry, and delights in watching them eat and play. As he snuggled his face into the smallest kitten's gray fur, I realized that he was able to completely relate to an animal for the first time.

I love watching him dance to the videos on television. I love watching him swing his arms wide in rhythm with the music. I love watching him jump, deliberately in beat with the music. I love seeing him glance my way to make sure that I am watching him as he imitates the video—the things we take for granted when we have "normal" children.

Photos had been particularly difficult since Benjamin had been about two years old. He appeared to have no understanding of the whole process of taking pictures. Looking at the camera was foreign to him as he squirmed to escape the clutches of whoever was unfortunate enough to have the task of holding him. Not long after his fourth birthday, on the day that school photos were taken, I asked Benjamin if he could please sit still and look at the camera so the photographer could take a good photo. I had a pleasant surprise when I picked him up at school that day.

"Benjamin did great today when his picture was taken," his teacher said.

"Really?" I exclaimed. "Did he hold still and actually look at the camera?"

"Yes, he really did."

At four years old, Benjamin's life is very different from even a year previously. He still gets up and watches whatever is on television, provided he isn't playing with one of his electronic toys. When I tell him it is time to get dressed for school, he dutifully follows me into his bedroom and grabs his notebook containing the photos of him dressing. He flips to the first page and points to the first picture, saying, "pants off." He then performs that task. He continues on to the next page, saying the activity, then performing it. After dressing, we go to the bathroom for hair and teeth brushing. He no longer winces as I brush his teeth. He admires himself as he gazes into the mirror while I brush his hair. He glances at me in the mirror, grinning when he sees me watching him.

"I need a big hug," I say as we finish.

"Big hug," he says as he grabs me forcefully, wrapping his arms and hands around my body, squeezing tightly.

"Time to get your backpack and go to school," I say.

He walks into the kitchen and grabs his backpack, slinging it over his shoulder. We begin our short walk to the school.

"Mailbox," he says as we walk down the sidewalk.

"Right," I say as we pass by it.

"Ride the train," he says as we pass the path that leads to the train station.

"First school, then ride train, if you have good behavior," I reply.

When we arrive at his classroom, he looks directly at his teacher and says, "Hi," placing his backpack in his designated cubby.

"Bye, Benjamin," I say, as I head toward the door.

"Bye, Momma," he replies, and he runs to the step stool to peek out the classroom window to watch as I leave.

When I arrive to pick him up, he runs to his cubby and slings his backpack over his shoulder.

"Hi, baby," I say.

"Hi, Momma," he replies.

As I talk to his teacher about his day, he waits patiently, knowing that our discussion will end quickly. As we talk, he turns back toward the door.

"Bye, Trisha. Bye, Pablo," he says to his classmates.

"You don't know how much time we put into teaching our children to do that, and Benjamin just does it," his teacher says, tears welling up in her eyes.

"I know, he amazes us every day," I reply, trying to hold back the tears. "How was his behavior today?"

"Wonderful."

"Great. I guess we'll get to go ride the train," I say.

Walking along the narrow sidewalk toward home, a yellow butterfly floats across our path. Benjamin immediately notices it and begins following it.

"Fickafly," he says, as it playfully flits in and out of the juniper bushes.

Benjamin follows its every move. It flies up the driveway, toward a neighbor's front door. He follows it until it turns abruptly, once again following the sidewalk path. The butterfly leads us all the way to our front door, then swiftly rises and disappears up into the clouds. Once we are inside, Benjamin eats his favorite meal, a gardenburger on five-grain bread, with avocado, onion, and french fries. Sometimes he gets distracted as he counts the french fries out loud, over and over again.

As we walk to the train station, Benjamin sings, "Five 'ittle 'ucks went ow one day, over the 'ills an' far away," the melody more perfect than the enunciation of the words, but definitely getting the point across.

I hear an airplane and look toward the sky. "Look, Benjamin, look at the airplane," I say, pointing skyward.

He looks at me, then to where I am pointing. He points at the sky, and repeats "airplane."

At the station, he boards the train when it arrives and runs to his favorite position at the back of the elevated platform. He points to a sign on the panel directly in front of his seat and reads, "Watch your step." He sits on his knees in the seat facing the window while we whiz past places with names like Dot Com Café and Bad Boys Bail Bonds. As we approach a station, he repeats the station name to himself. He is totally engrossed in the experience, getting excited as the train approaches each station, knowing that the doors will soon open, then shut.

As we reach our station, he jumps up, but waits patiently as an elderly woman descends the stairs in front of us. We walk to the ice cream shop, where he selects his flavor, either "strawburry" or "mint." Sometimes he asks for "both." He sits in the park and carefully eats the ice cream. I never get tired of seeing him eat ice cream. When we first learned of his milk allergy, my husband had been devastated, thinking that he would never be able to eat an ice cream cone. Now, he eats one every day. Benjamin stands up and throws the remainder of the cone and the well-used napkins in the trash.

We continue down the street to the music store. We stop at the corner and he presses the button, waiting for the "walking man" that indicates it is safe to cross the street. We cross the street, and Benjamin runs up to the front window of the music store, pointing. He taps his finger on the glass, saying "cello," then "violin," continuing on until he has identified all of the several dozen musical instruments in the window. Then we continue on to the bakery, where he goes inside to look at the heart, turtle, and cat-shaped cookies. Sometimes we buy a cookie, sometimes we don't. He doesn't get upset either way. A change in routine without a tantrum, especially involving something that he loves to eat, is a huge milestone for him.

We follow our route back to the train, board, and ride the train until we reach our stop. He runs off the train onto the platform, stopping directly across from the first set of wheels. He "stims," watching the front wheels of the first car as the train leaves the station, then glances back at the wheels of the second car. He stands transfixed and "stimming" until the train is no longer in sight. We walk back to our house, holding hands when crossing the street. Arriving at the house, he either heads to the backyard to ride his tricycle, or watches Wiggles videos.

When he hears a friend's car in the driveway, he runs to our front gate saying, "Hi, Meleessa." He has progressed from calling her "Mss" to "Missa" to "Meleessa," and occasionally calls her "sweetheart" because she often calls him this.

We venture out to the local wholesale warehouse store. He seems to have difficulty with the crowd, but manages to maintain himself. He shouts out occasionally, but my instructions to have a quiet mouth are successful, until we reach the checkout area. He is perfectly content sitting in the front of the basket, until the checker grabs the basket, getting within inches of his body. Immediately, he starts crying and trying to get out of the basket. Like a wild animal trapped in a corner, he obviously wants to get away from her.

"It's okay, Benjamin, it's okay," I say, trying to get him to make eye contact with me.

He finally looks in my direction and starts to calm down as the checker moves away from him.

"I know the lady got in your space," I say, as we walk to our car. "I'm sorry she got too close." He is perfectly calm now.

Sometimes he runs into the room roaring like a lion. I know that this is my cue to start chasing him all over the house. I am more than happy to oblige. I hide somewhere in the house, and he tries to find me. When he does, I jump out and chase him, as he giggles and shouts mock screams until I am too exhausted to run anymore. His body jumps and reacts when I lunge from behind the door, but he is never afraid.

Shortly after Ben's fifth birthday, we had an opportunity to move to South Australia. Ben delights in the wildlife and abundance of nature here. He races up hiking trails past waterfalls as cockatiels fly overhead. We make weekly visits to the ocean where he jumps in the surf and "stims" on the waves. His sleeping patterns have greatly improved. Ben will eat a wider selection of fruits and vegetables, and occasionally eats meat. He can sometimes ask for what he wants in complete sentences. I've noticed that he is able to say what he is thinking. When he gets stuck on a computer game, he says, "Computer is not working." When he is looking for me, I hear him say, "Where's Mommy?" Since Benjamin has been on the dairy/gluten-free, low-salicylate, additive-free diet, we've even discovered that he has a great sense of humor and a penchant for Rod Stewart music. His teacher reports that he has become very affectionate with the school staff and says that he is just as easy to care for as the "normal" peers in his preschool class.

Each day I look forward to receiving what I have named my "Benjamin fix." Benjamin exudes that puppy dog excitement and capacity for unconditional love, but with much greater depth and intensity. I first experienced this nothing-held-back kind of love in my vision of "the master," but I can reach out and hold this little master anytime I want or need him. By kissing a hand, touching a face, or offering a hug, Benjamin often extends this loving feeling to friends and family now, usually when they are in particular need of it.

His father usually takes him to the park in the evenings. He loves to swing and run up and down the tall slide, trying to coax his father to follow him up the winding stairs.

Near bedtime, he comes to me saying, "Brush teeth," and takes my hand to lead me to the bathroom. He races to the rocking chair saying, "Rock," to indicate that he is ready for bed. I still rock him to sleep at night and slip him in between his crisp sheets covered with frogs, jumping and sitting on lily pads. Now he is actually aware of the little frogs dancing playfully there.

14 The Judgment

You are unconditioned spirit that's trapped in conditions like the sun in eclipse.

—Jelaluddin Rumi

From the moment I laid eyes on my little boy, I was filled with an overwhelming sense of awareness that he possessed a certain depth, that he carried a special secret, like a pearl buried in the oyster, waiting to be discovered. As if to punctuate this feeling, more than a dozen times in his short life total strangers have approached me to tell me that there was "something special about that little boy."

Even when I was in deep despair after his diagnosis, I was acutely aware that some burdens were his alone to bear. I knew that it was not my job to save him from all difficulty. My job was not to "rescue" him from autism. I was all too aware that my own personal growth seemed to occur only after a high price had been exacted in the form of some difficulty that I was forced to overcome. Many times I prayed that I could help him, but only enough to remove any obstacles that might interfere with whatever it was that he came into the world to accomplish. Many times I faced the possibility that he would never speak or communicate beyond the level where he was. I not only faced that possibility, but was somehow able to bring myself to accept it.

The more time I spent alone with my little boy, watching and observing him over the course of many months, I began to realize that his world wasn't a "bad" one. Even when he seemed to be "lost" in his own world, I was struck by the fact that sometimes I longed to be "lost" with him. His world seemed, at times, much more preferable than mine. The "bad" part was the world's expectations about how he should act and what he should be doing and how he should be doing it. Donna Williams explains:

> As people began to explain how other people experienced my behavior, I came to learn that all behavior had two definitions: theirs and mine. These "helpful" people were trying to help me to "overcome my ignorance" yet they never tried to understand the way I saw the world. It seemed so simple to them. There were rules. The rules were right. I obviously needed their help to learn them.[1]

In the face of constant threats of institutionalization, Donna Williams found that:

> It was this fear of having "my own world" taken away from me that resulted in behavior that forced me to deny "my own world" in place of a more presentable, well-mannered, sociable, though emotionless shell. "They" never got to lay a hand on the real me, but more and more, to their elation, I began to stop visiting myself. I began to stop looking at the spots and losing myself in the colors. I began to lose a grip on my love of the things around me and, in doing so, was left with "their" shallow securities and complete lack of guarantees. My hatred became my only realness, and when I was not angry, I said sorry for breathing, for taking up space, and even began to say sorry for saying sorry. This total denial of a right to live was a consequence of learning to act normal. Everything outside of me told me that my survival was to rest on my refining the act of acting normal. On the inside I knew that by definition this meant that whatever and whoever I was naturally was unworthy of acceptance, belonging or even life.[2]

I was all too aware of this need to act normal, to fit in, to be accepted. I knew how dangerous it could be to break that rule. People might just as well be wearing huge signs in bold-face letters plastered on their chests reading, **"Don't tread on my reality."** Like Donna Williams, I knew that "people think of reality as some sort of guarantee they can rely on." Yet, from her earliest memories she states she could remember finding her "only dependable security was in losing all awareness of the things usually considered real." In doing this, she was able to "lose all sense of self."[3]

Perhaps this was the awareness of Shams of Tabriz, friend and spiritual guide to Jelaluddin Rumi, when he said that "people say that human beings are microcosms and this outer universe a macrocosm, but for us the outer is a tiny wholeness and the inner life the vast reality."[4]

Individuals spend years practicing meditation and seeking the advice of gurus, with the ultimate goal of being able to lose all sense of self, to "achieve inner peace and tranquility."[5] I, too, have worked hard to finally quiet the words, "I'm not good enough, I'm not good enough," racing through my mind, each time searing the pain deeper and deeper into my psyche. My salvation comes in those moments of feeling truly connected.

I've learned to achieve grounding by watching my son as he communes with nature. I've learned to bring the knowledge of my soul into my body, allowing my physical and my emotional body to speak freely to me. I have learned to be fully grounded in my body, experiencing spirit and flesh at the same time. I've learned from my son's struggle to be grounded in material reality. His battle was to stay in his physical body and experience his life from a bodily perspective. Mine was to stop focusing on material reality and to reexperience those things not locked in time at all, those things that exist now, then, forever, wherever. My challenge was to find the focus of awareness where Benjamin lived, and intellectually to screen my experiences there for their potential relevance and usefulness to physical existence. Benjamin and I are both learning the same skills, just approaching our perceived deficiencies from different ends of the spectrum, each of us striving to be whole.

Donna Williams states:

> In the world, the emphasis is on complexity, yet it is misleading to believe that complexity cannot be found in simplicity. People who pride themselves on the ability to think complexly with their conscious mind often still have not found the ability to think in symbols with their subconscious mind. In this blind self-assurance, so many attempts are made by well-meaning people to drag children's consciousness into the so-called complexities of "the world" without first asking to what extent that world is worthy of them. Perhaps this is the real madness, naiveté, and ignorance.[6]

Perhaps the words I perceived in one of my morning meditations served as a warning: "There is no need to dumb Benjamin down to your level of awareness."

15 The Realization

Believe in your children.
—*response by Tito Mukhopadhyay, a 14-year-old autistic boy when asked for his advice to parents of autistic children*[1]

Once, my husband and I fantasized about how simple our lives would have been if we had two normal children. Some things would have been so much simpler. There would have been no need to keep such close tabs on Benjamin. I could have relaxed and chatted with someone while at the playground. We could have eaten out in restaurants. We could have taken trips to anyplace we desired. Our houses, cars, schools, and where we live wouldn't have had to be carefully selected to meet Benjamin's needs. We could have kept playing out our lives, totally unaware that there was any other way of being.

We would be living in the same town, doing the same things, working the same jobs, and repeating the same pointless patterns in our lives. We would be playing it safe, doing what we had been told to do in order to be in control of our lives. We would not be taking chances. We would be living the plan that was set out for us generations ago. We would never have known anything different if it weren't for Benjamin.

We would never have had the courage to move halfway across the country and then halfway around the world for certain schools and better climate. We never would have known how well our daughter would have done in her new school. We never would have seen the joy in Benjamin's eyes when he first looked a kangaroo in the eyes or seen Karis hold a koala in her arms. We never would have known that our daughter could make such an astounding connection with nature.

My husband and I would never have known what it was like to trust each other enough to take these risks. We wouldn't have known how this trust would make our relationship even stronger. We never would have known that such an amazing force could take charge of our lives and guide us on our path in perfect synchronicity. We never would have known the joy of risking everything and of gaining everything. We realize that we wouldn't change a thing.

I know that I was prepared for Benjamin at every step of the way. Every person that I needed to help me was there, waiting for me. My meditation classes that I began attending during the month he was conceived, the therapists who appeared in our home at exactly the right moments, the helpers who were brought into my life to make me feel secure in working with Benjamin, the wonderful teachers and therapists who all played their parts in perfect synchronicity, Donna Williams; they were all there. All I had to do was ask, and it was delivered. How many of us go along in life, never asking, hoping, or daring to dream for anything to be different?

Benjamin and I have a close bond that is difficult to express in words. We were two people who spoke different languages, trapped on a sinking ship, about to drown in the sea of our situation. Neither of us knew if we were going to make it, but we have, and we are both changed because of it.

I realize that if it weren't for his condition, I would never have known him the way that I do. Without verbal language, I was forced to watch, observe, and see what wasn't obvious. Without the usual body clues, I had to get into his mind, try to read his thoughts, and attempt to feel what he was feeling. Trapped in a small body with no way of communicating with the rest of the world, he was at the mercy of the situation. He was the one with no control. He had to trust that everything would be all right, that we would figure it out. He was the brave one. He was my best teacher.

Kahlil Gibran, in *The Prophet,* states: "The teacher who walks in the shadow of the temple, among his followers, gives not of his wisdom but rather of his faith and his lovingness. If he is indeed wise he does not bid you enter the house of his wisdom, but rather leads you to the threshold of your own mind."[2]

Benjamin has taken me to that threshold, and gently lifted me over it. In the shadow of Benjamin's unconditional love, I learned to love and accept, without expecting anything in return. I began to understand that it was not up to my husband or my children to change to fit my expectations. My family and my possessions could never make me happy. Happiness, in the face of whatever life had in store for me, was my responsibility. Benjamin demonstrated that living each day, exacting the richness in each moment, was how to truly experience life.

With the help of many others, I feel I can humbly begin to answer the question, "Where was Benjamin?" The answer is that he has been right here all the time, just living in a much different, more expanded way—a way I am just beginning to understand and experience. He is the boy between two worlds. In one world he possesses a sensitive body that feels too much, that normal things harm, and that traditional methods fail. In the other "speeded up" world of light, sparkling color particles, blocks of color, and patterns of energy fields, he allows us to glimpse a realm much deeper, richer, and far more wondrous than most of us can imagine, a world of unconditional love, healing, and pure experience. From this place he asks us not to "fix" him, but beckons us to join him. He encourages us to experience what he has already mastered, to love and accept ourselves, just the way we are.

Whispers

Shhhhhhhhhh!
Come close and
I'll tell you a secret!
About the blessing and the curse
Of being born
A Clear-seeing child.
There was no gain in outward aggression
Nor causing others pain.
Passivity was the safer harbor
Revenge never sweetly won.
Whatever I created in that vein,
I was also forced to endure.
Through extraordinary sensory means,
The pain of others
At once became my own.
And the blessing?
Can you guess it?
I met myself at every turn.

—*Rabyn Judith Pillsbury*

PART II

For Parents and Caregivers

16 The Things That Work

Everything I need to know is revealed to me. Everything I need
comes to me.
All is well in my life.

—Lousie L. Hay

Nature and Grounding

From the moment that Benjamin began to walk, he had a profound love of nature and the outdoors. His favorite activity was to
strip off his shoes and run barefooted in our backyard. A look of bliss
on his face, he would run endlessly back and forth. I know now that
running barefooted in the grass is an excellent way of grounding,
which is the act of connecting one's life energy to the energy of the
earth. Grounding increases the electromagnetic energy in the lower
body.

I also discovered that certain foods help accomplish grounding,
including Benjamin's much loved fast-food french fries. The salt and
grease help bring the body energies down into the lower chakras.[1]
Autistic children's craving for fast-food fries is legendary. Their craving
for these greasy treats may simply be an attempt to get their focus of
awareness back into the body. Grounding helps to relieve imbalances

caused by electromagnetic and geomagnetic disturbances when shifting from "higher dimensions into lower ones."[2] These disturbances may cause feelings of "distress or moodiness."[3]

Often, Benjamin would stray from our carefully manicured lawn. I would always find him standing barefooted beneath one of the two giant oak trees in our backyard. With outstretched arms he would stand beneath the trees. Before I had an understanding of why he preferred to be near these giant trees, I would complain to my husband that we had a beautiful lawn with a rose arbor and a fountain, and I would always find Benjamin in the rough, shoeless and hugging the trees. One day when he was still nonverbal, I found him standing beneath one of the trees, and I scooped him up and asked him what he was doing out there. He looked into my eyes, leaned over, and hugged the trunk of the oak tree. It was as if he were hugging a favorite friend. This behavior was notable, since at that time, his hugs were usually reserved for me. Trees seem to structure direct earth vibrations to create their own energy matrix,[4] and it is likely this energy that Benjamin was sensing.

Children instinctively know how to use nature to ground. Their reluctance to wear shoes, their desire to run barefooted in the grass, climb the nearest tree, and be outdoors is evidence of such knowledge. Too soon, this connection with nature is replaced with classrooms and sterile office environments. Their natural grounding ability is lost and with it comes a life lived in an ungrounded state, with the electromagnetic energy descending no further than head or chest level. Most adults typically live life in their heads. Children live in a more grounded state, until they are told to get serious with life. As an adult, living life in a grounded state "requires the willingness, honesty and courage to face ourselves as we are and our world as it is—no distance, no exclusions, no avoidances, no anesthesia."[5] It is living life at the bone.

When Benjamin was almost two years old, we took a family trip to Charleston, South Carolina. Benjamin experienced the ocean for the first time. He ran toward the surf, then turned around and ran away from it. He seemed to be truly happy there. I made the comment to my husband that at some point we would have to live somewhere near the ocean while Benjamin was growing up. Since our move to Australia, we make frequent trips to the ocean.

Benjamin stands in the surf, jumping up and down, a look of total bliss on his angelic face. He actually seems to sense the energy of the waves and knows where they will break, moving to a position closer or farther from each wave, so that the water level where he is standing remains constant. He likes the water to come up to just past his knees, so he predicts and adjusts his distance to accomplish this. I have watched him do this for hours at a time, afraid for his safety when he gets close to a large wave as it breaks, only to watch the wave collapse on itself as the water travels toward him at knee level. The only time he gets taken by surprise is when he becomes distracted and bends over to "stim" on the energy of the wave. His sensing of the energy of the water overcomes any other awareness at that time, and he typically ends up wet and choking from the spray of the surf.

I believe that it is no coincidence that Benjamin's favorite activities are running barefooted in the grass, hugging trees, playing in the surf, and eating french fries; these are all activities that are known to result in grounding or to increase the body's energy field. I believe that in the days of his worst physical health, his constant running was a futile attempt to ground himself, to bring his awareness back into his physical body.

Learning Techniques

Electronic learning toys fascinate Benjamin. We bought him a Leap's Phonics Pond by Leap Frog. When he pressed the letters of the alphabet on the front of the toy, he could hear the sound of each letter. He played with the toy one weekend, and the next day he identified each letter of the magnetic alphabet on our refrigerator door, even when we rearranged them. Later he used the same toy to teach himself the sounds associated with each letter of the alphabet. We bought him a Leap Pad Learning System by Leap Frog.[6] His favorite Leap Frog book is *Music: Classical Composers and Their Greatest Hits*. He loves hearing the individual musical instruments, and has learned the names of each instrument. The toy is wonderful because it allows him to choose and play musical selections when he wants to hear them.

Benjamin loves music, and it is a big motivator for his learning. He loves all of the videos by the Wiggles, an Australian group that produces children's videos.[7] The videos are very musical, and have lots of dancing and movement. Benjamin began interacting with the videos before interacting with most people. The videos are primarily musical and are so fun and engaging that he got drawn into them. For households with children of differing ages, the Wiggles videos are some of the few videos that my older daughter will watch with Benjamin, which eliminates disagreements over what to watch.

Another video Benjamin loves because it contains two of his most favorite things, trains and music, is *I Love Toy Trains—The Music Video*.[8] He never tires of watching this video, and it holds his attention for a full half-hour.

While in a bookstore recently, my daughter selected *The Alley Cat's Meow*[9] from the numerous children's books on display and handed it to my husband to purchase. My husband's first instinct was to put it back on the shelf. Then he noticed that it was written by Kathi Appelt, a dear friend of ours from Texas. He purchased the book and it quickly became one of Benjamin's favorites. In its beautifully illustrated pages, it combines three of Benjamin's favorite things: cats, trains, and dancing.

Toilet Training

Since autistic children generally find it difficult to understand verbal instructions and linear sequences, the most important tools that a parent of an autistic child can own are a digital camera and a color printer. I stumbled upon the idea of making visual images for things that I needed Benjamin to do when we were attempting to toilet-train him. He was extremely successful with urinating in the toilet using the following protocols. Within two days, he was consistently using the toilet for urinating.

We had much more difficulty with him eliminating in the toilet. For several months, I cleaned him after accidents. One day, his in-home trainer suggested that we use what is commonly referred to as a "social story" for his toileting procedure. She took digital photos of the potty, Benjamin pulling down his pants, then sitting on the potty, then pulling up his pants, and flushing the potty. She then took a photo of the "evidence" of using the potty and paired it with a candy wrapper to represent his chosen reward. He reviewed the pictures in sequence in a folder for a day. The next day he eliminated in the potty and he was trained.

I believe that unlike urinating in the potty, which is self-reinforcing for a boy, it was difficult for him to understand eliminating in the potty because he couldn't actually see himself doing it. Once he was able to get the picture of the sequence in his head, he was able to follow the procedure every time without fail.

Benjamin's first teacher, Janet Boutton, uses a method of toilet training that has never failed to train the numerous autistic children that she has taught over the years. Her method involves putting a child in regular underwear and regularly sitting the child on the toilet at timed intervals. Her method, the Toilet Training Protocol, appears in appendix A.

Behavioral Difficulties

Benjamin's understanding of discipline is very different from our daughter's. When dealing with Karis, I could explain what behaviors were expected, and she usually complied. If she didn't, she knew what she was supposed to be doing and an appropriate consequence quickly followed.

I soon learned that any methods I had used with Karis failed miserably with Benjamin. He just didn't seem to "get" what it was I was trying to get across. If I told Benjamin not to do something, such as repeatedly opening and shutting a door, he would fuss when I corrected him, then just go right back to the same behavior. I began to realize that Benjamin was a visual learner. For some reason, verbal instructions were extremely difficult for him to understand.

Sometimes redirecting him to a more appropriate activity would be successful. Just stopping the behavior didn't seem to help him find a more appropriate activity. I would have to take Benjamin physically to an acceptable activity or bring the activity to him. If redirecting failed after several attempts, I used two poster boards for displaying different behaviors that I term "good" or "bad" behaviors. At the top of the poster board I wrote in bold letters either "Good Behavior" or "Bad Behavior." I took digital photos of Benjamin crying, fussing, screaming, kicking, and whining, and printed them out on a color printer. Then I did the same with a picture of Benjamin crying in his room. The pictures are attached to the poster board and underneath each picture I wrote the word that describes the behavior.

Benjamin is allowed to engage in these behaviors only in his room. If Benjamin engages in these behaviors other than in his room, he is taken into his room and shown the poster board. Then I verbally say each "bad" behavior out loud, then finish by saying "bad behavior in Ben's room. When you are finished with bad behavior, you can come out of your room." The pictures enabled him to form a picture in his mind that he could grasp.

I repeated the same process with "good" behavior by snapping photos of Benjamin smiling, laughing, hugging, playing quietly, sitting down, and so forth. After I finish saying the "bad" behaviors, I say "good behaviors are smiling, sitting quietly, laughing, playing quietly, sitting still. If you have good behavior today, we'll go ride the train or go to the park," or whatever activity I can take him to that day.

A list of the charts I created for Benjamin appears in appendix B.

I believe that it is important to address behaviors as they occur, rather than try to condition a child in an artificially created environment, such as behavior modification discrete trials. In a natural setting, the child is dealing with the natural emotion of the situation, not the added stress of being forced to focus continually on what someone else decides is important at that moment.

We made "social story" books for any situation that proved to be stressful to Benjamin. We had traveled many times with Benjamin on an airplane before using this technique. I can say it was complete and total chaos. He ended up screaming for almost the entire trip, much to our dismay and the dismay of everyone else on the plane. We used a social story for the plane trip when we moved to California. Previously, we had taken photos of every stage of the trip, including the arrival at the airport, walking to the gate, waiting at the gate, walking onto the plane, sitting in the seat, playing with the toys we would bring with us on the trip, eating his snacks, drinking his juice, reading his books, and listening to his tapes.

This requires a little bit of creativity, since someone must make a similar trip so that photos can be taken for the book. I've asked many kind strangers to snap photos of me at every stage of an airplane trip. I believe one of the most important photos was of me sitting in the seat next to an empty chair. For this photo I would tell Benjamin, "This is where you will sit quietly next to Momma."

These children do not understand linear sequence, and airplane travel involves many linear steps. Benjamin reviewed his travel "social story" for several days before the trip and did wonderfully on the long trip to California. No one even knew there was a child sitting next to me until he saw that we were starting to land, then he started to get excited and antsy to exit the plane. I was amazed at the difference in his behavior. The photos gave him an overall sequence of events in the form of images that he could hold onto in his mind. Any time we are going to engage in an activity that Benjamin is not familiar with, I go over the sequence with Benjamin in advance, and this greatly increases the odds of a successful outing. If it involves many steps, I create a social story that he can physically look at before the outing.

I review "first, then" sequences with Benjamin many times each day. First we must eat lunch, then we can ride the train. First we go to the store, then we can go to the park. First we go to school, then we ride the train. He has to be reminded over and over again that our world occurs in a linear sequence. Sometimes he is just too focused on something to switch to something else. During these episodes, the only technique that I have found is to redirect his behavior into something more appropriate. If he wants to open and shut a door repeatedly, just to watch it open and shut, I usually have to redirect his attention. The activity is so attractive to him that simply telling him not to do it isn't always effective.

Many times each day I have to remind Benjamin to use language to tell me what he needs. I constantly tap my chin, asking him to "use words" to tell me what he wants. When he fusses or pulls on my arm, I say, "I want . . ." then wait for his response. I force him into unfamiliar territory, over and over again, making him use words to express himself.

Sometimes, when Benjamin gets fussy for no apparent reason, I mirror his behavior. I fuss back at him. Able to understand the visual appearance of his inappropriate behavior, a sudden shift results, and Benjamin begins to laugh. He explodes in deep, loud belly laughs and he is able to shift into more appropriate behavior. I must admit that I have thrown myself on the floor before in a full-blown, pretend temper tantrum, mirroring his behavior. Of course, this method is difficult to use when other people are present, but I did use this method one day when Benjamin was very fussy and uncooperative when we were walking down a crowded street. My admonitions to stop the behavior were ineffective. I stopped and stood him on a bench, so that we were at eye level. I began to fuss and whine, just as he was doing. He immediately began to laugh. Once he was calm, I explained that he was about to lose his train privileges for the next day. I asked him if he could have good behavior, and he replied "yes." We continued on our way with him displaying excellent behavior for the rest of the day.

I believe the reason this works is due to energy field interaction. The normal response to a child's temper tantrum is a negative emotion experienced by the parent, which results in a negative shift in the parent's energy field. It is a perfectly normal response to become furious that you can't even finish your grocery shopping because of your child's behavior. These emotions will affect the child, however, since we know that even plants respond positively or negatively to strong emotions.[10] Emotions arise from an altered electromagnetic environment, and temporarily restructure the electromagnetic field.[11] This interaction is why Benjamin was mirroring my moods. If I became angry, he became even more angry. If I stopped myself before I became angry and demonstrated a more positive energy, then he became more balanced and exhibited more positive behavior.

Once, while standing at a street corner waiting for a light to change, Benjamin and I witnessed a driver become very angry and agitated toward a driver waiting for traffic in order to make a left turn. The second driver cursed, yelled, and motioned to the driver in front of her, trying to make the first driver get out of her way. Benjamin immediately became emotional and started trying to get away from the situation by running into the oncoming traffic. The more she yelled, the more he tried to get away from her.

I was reminded of the old Steve Martin skit where he gets "happy feet." All of a sudden, it is as if his feet had volition of their own, moving wildly, almost out of control. His happy feet just wanted to get him out of there. In this situation, I stopped at the nearest safe place, holding Benjamin and talking softly to him until he was able to calm down. I focus on my own level of calm, knowing that my state of mind is directly influencing his. I immediately attempt to put myself into a calm, meditative state while talking to him. This does require practice, since initially my body immediately responded in a negative fashion when Benjamin had inappropriate behavior. I've found that the calmer I am, the more responsive he is and the quicker he is able to bring himself under control.

Body Discomfort

Benjamin enjoys any type of massage. He loves lotions applied to his hands, feet, back, chest, and legs. Even when he was experiencing great body discomfort in the early days of his diagnosis, massage was always comforting to him. His grandmother would lovingly apply lotions after his bath, and these massages helped to calm him.

Sometimes when Benjamin seems to be particularly stressed or out of balance, I quickly place him into a lukewarm bath. The bath works instantly to change his mood, perhaps increasing the negative ions in his energy field. Sometimes I add a drop of an aromatherapy oil, such as lavender, to increase the bath's calming effect. I've followed Dr. Pouls' suggestion outlined in *The Natural Medicine Guide to Autism,* to place Benjamin in Epsom salt baths.[12] The baths seem to produce a calming effect that lasts for an entire day. Sometimes autistic children have difficulty absorbing magnesium in the gastrointestinal tract. The baths provide an alternate way to get magnesium into the system. She suggests adding a half to a full cup of Epsom salts to a tub of warm water, as warm as the child can handle. The child should soak for 15 or 20 minutes. The baths may be given daily. The magnesium actually helps to relax the child's muscles and serves to gently detoxify the body, drawing toxins out through the skin.

In the early days, we often put a padded, weighted vest on Benjamin. These vests apply slight pressure on the body, which helps to calm the nervous system. We borrowed one from his school to use at home.

Benjamin responds very favorably to certain kinds of music. Music is believed to promote healing through the vibrational energy of different tones or pitches of sound, bringing the tissues and organs of the body into harmony. The selection that has proven to have the most calming effect on his physical body is *Seven Metals, Singing Bowls of Tibet* by Benjamin Iobst.[13] No matter how excited Benjamin may be, when this selection is played, he becomes quiet and still, listening to the music. The selection was created by a bodywork therapist for use in his practice and was designed for deep meditation and relaxation.

A tape that has a calming effect on both of my children is *Macaroni Pony,*[14] produced by the Achates Corporation. The tape is a blending of soft, precisely sequenced sound patterns with a scripted story. This tape was one Benjamin used successfully on the airplane during our trip to California. Two other favorites are *Robbie the Rabbit,*[15] and *Joy Jumper,*[16] produced by The Monroe Institute. The stories, along with nature sounds and Hemi-Sync frequencies, have a very calming and soothing effect. Hemi-Sync sound patterns help achieve and sustain synchronized brain-wave activity in both hemispheres of the brain. *Joy Jumper* contains a bedtime story on track one and music on track two. I find the music track very relaxing and often listen to it myself to relieve stress.

Riding the light rail train has a very calming effect on Benjamin. An interesting note is that the train operates on direct current (DC) electricity, not on alternating current (AC). DC is continuous electric current, perhaps serving to boost Benjamin's electromagnetic field. Another factor may be that most people riding the train are simply *being,* not *doing,* so they are simply letting their minds idle, allowing themselves to relax. In this state, strong negative emotions are not present, so there would be no attendant emotions to trigger a response in Benjamin, except in the case of a person who is emotionally unbalanced.

Illness

When Benjamin becomes ill, we use natural medicine treatments to help his body heal and balance itself. We have found that these techniques work for the entire family, and we very rarely seek treatment through conventional medicine. I have learned very basic Lymph Drainage techniques, which I begin using at the first signs of illness. I also use various methods of balancing the body at this time, including basic CranioSacral Therapy techniques and energy balancing. The duration of our illnesses is typically about a day. I have also used homeopathic treatments with great success.

Discipline

Early on, one of the most difficult things about Benjamin's condition was that we were unsure of how much Benjamin understood. Consequently, he was allowed to exhibit behaviors that we never would have permitted had he been a "normal" child. He developed a habit of lying on the floor and kicking the door when he wanted to go outside or when he was sent to his room for uncontrollable crying. I tried everything to let him know that this behavior was unacceptable. My yelling at him to stop kicking and my exasperated state left Benjamin in tears and were totally ineffective.

Finally, the school district's in-home trainer suggested that he might be demonstrating that behavior to get attention. Get attention, I thought. He has my undivided attention virtually 24 hours a day. I decided to give her suggestion a try. When he kicked the door, we would walk to the door and say "no kicking, kicking is bad behavior," then walk away. Sometimes if he was in the room with us, we would hold his feet for a few seconds. If he continued to kick, we would simply ignore him altogether. After a few days, he discovered that he no longer could get our immediate attention with this behavior, and much to our relief, he stopped doing it. One of the most difficult things I have ever done is to stand by and let Benjamin kick the door as hard as he was physically able to kick. I now believe that by my not reacting negatively to his emotional state—walking away—he was able to bring himself under control much more quickly.

Once he began communicating, he demonstrated behaviors that were similar to a two-year-old child's behavior. He stretched his boundaries again and again. There are two reasons that it is very tempting as a parent to allow bad behavior in these children. The first being that it can be very difficult to discipline an autistic child with limited communication skills. Discipline is difficult when you have no feedback from a child that he or she understands why the behavior is unacceptable. When there is limited communication, it requires a great leap of faith on the parent's part that the child understands. Benjamin would lose the privilege of riding the train for bad behavior, long before he could actually communicate that he understood why he was losing a privilege. Several months into the more strict behavior regimen, I was greatly relieved when Benjamin shouted, "Oh, no!" when I pointed out that his bad behavior was about to result in the loss of his train privileges for the next day.

Another complicating factor is that Benjamin's reactions could be so much more explosive and out of control than any behaviors that our daughter ever demonstrated. He could become so fixated on something that it seemed that changing his focus, much less hoping for some understanding of why the situation was unacceptable, seemed almost impossible at times. I found that explaining any variations in routine in advance greatly increased the odds of acceptable behavior. Often if the difference in routine was substantial, I would repeat the same information four or five times, using the "first we do X, then we do Y" method.

I've thought a great deal about the children whom I prosecuted during my tenure as juvenile prosecutor. Most of the children I dealt with seemed to have unresolved physical or emotional problems and a total lack of personal boundaries. Boundaries are "distinguishing and keeping out what is not me, and holding in place what is."[17] I know that trying to discipline Benjamin before the problems with his physical body were resolved was as pointless as flying a kite in a hurricane. Everyone just ended up crashing and burning. I wondered if the parents of these children were just completely overwhelmed by their children. I certainly could relate to that feeling. Many parents were either absent, so overwhelmed in their own lives that they were unwilling or unable to deal with the behaviors, or extremely permissive due to the parents' desire not to re-create the harshness of their own childhoods. Usually, the patterns began in early childhood. I noticed a consistent pattern in virtually all cases. There seemed to be no consistent consequences for the child's aberrant behaviors. The child did not understand his or her own boundaries.

Charles Whitfield says, "A boundary or limit is how far we can comfortably go in a relationship and how far someone else can comfortably go with us. A boundary is not just a mental construct: Our boundaries are real. Other people's boundaries are real."[18]

Barbara Whitfield states, "Boundaries and limits serve a useful purpose: they protect the well-being and integrity of our True Self, our Child Within. Our awareness of boundaries and limits first helps us discover who we are. Until we know who we are, it will be difficult for us to have healthy relationships of any sort. Without an awareness of boundaries, it is difficult to sort out who is unsafe to be around, including people who are toxic for us and people who may mistreat or abuse us."[19]

If a child fails to learn boundaries from a parent, then society, the court system, or the school system will take over to teach those boundaries. Society fears the actions of people who lack boundaries and will operate to reduce its own fear level. Generally, the result will not be loving discipline for your child. I believe that it is very important to teach both of my children about proper boundaries. It is even more crucial to teach boundaries to sensitive children who are able to feel much of the pain and emotions of others. In learning about boundaries, they can distinguish whether what they are feeling is "theirs" or "someone else's."

My daughter is constantly being reminded that she can do anything that she wants to, provided that she is willing to suffer the consequences. The consequences of bad behavior come swiftly and surely. One way to traumatize your child emotionally is to respond inconsistently and arbitrarily to your child's behavior. When a child does something that they know is wrong, they are asking you to help define their boundaries. Not helping your child in this situation can be traumatic to the child. In a desperate attempt for clarity, the next attempt for a boundary definition is likely to occur in an even more dramatic context. All of us like knowing where the walls are. We like knowing that the people we trust will keep their word. If a parent reassures a frightened child that they will never leave the child, yet the parent is inconsistent and fails to follow through on their declarations on other occasions, then how does the child know that a parent "means it" when they say they will never leave?

Benjamin is expected not to damage items that belong to another. He is expected to pick up after himself, dress himself, and feed himself. He performs these duties because he is expected to. He is consistently and firmly reminded that these duties are his responsibility. The difficulty is in choosing your battles. With "normal" children, guilt and a certain level of fear can be used to control behaviors. Autistic children know nothing about guilt and do not relate in the same way to fear. Because Benjamin is so visual, the only successful method has been to use the charts to point out what is acceptable and unacceptable behavior, then pair those behaviors with appropriate consequences. If Benjamin has good behavior, he can go ride the train or go to the park. If he has bad behavior, then he loses his train or park privileges. We are constantly adding and updating the charts as the months progress.

17 Advice for Parents and Caregivers

In finding treatments for a child, the greatest guiding force should be your intuition. If you don't like or feel comfortable with a teacher or a therapist, then it's very likely that your child won't either. One speech therapist actually held Benjamin in her lap for most of the 30-minute session that took place in our home. She claimed that he had to "get used to her" so that he could learn. I wasn't comfortable with her asserting herself in his space, and judging by the shrill shrieks that were his only means of communication at that time, he was even less thrilled with her methodology. That therapist was asked not to return. Again, I had to ask myself, would someone do this to an adult? Of course they wouldn't. The therapist was frustrated and unsure of herself, so she decided that she would let him know who was in charge by attempting to assert control over the situation by forcing him to deal with her.

Don't be afraid or ashamed to talk to others about your child's condition. Use the word "autistic." Use it until it feels just like any other word coming from your lips. So many parents are afraid of labels. I'm sorry, but the world is already full of them; I don't think that one more is going to make that much more of a difference. We have no problem saying we're blond or brunette, or African-American or Norwegian. The only difference with calling someone "autistic" is the fear and shame that some associate with the condition. We're

151

afraid to call our children "autistic" because we fear the pity of others. We're afraid of admitting that our child isn't what society considers perfect. Facing that feeling will make it disappear, and it will become a nonissue. It is a case of not resisting "what is." I know that no matter what strides Benjamin makes toward a "normal" life, he will never be normal, and that is fine by me. We have many people with what are considered normal capabilities, but what the world needs are visionaries, people that can think outside the box and stretch us beyond what we know right now. Our striving for normalcy is what keeps us stuck where we are.

I have found that telling people that Benjamin is autistic has had some fairly amazing results. When I tell someone about Benjamin's condition, usually it is because of some behavior or situation that he cannot tolerate. There are so many children being diagnosed with autism spectrum disorders that everyone seems to know someone who has a child with the condition. A great deal of information is exchanged that is helpful either to me, or to someone else. The second thing that usually happens is that people in the situation immediately change their attitude and become extremely helpful. We have a lot of conditioning in our society that if a child is misbehaving in public, then it is the fault of the parent, who has failed to provide appropriate discipline and guidance.

People make judgments based on their past experience in similar situations. Most people have never had close interactions with a child like Benjamin, so it is unreasonable for me to expect anyone to understand him. Before Benjamin entered our lives, I had never seen a child who refused to wait in a line or known that there were children who could instantly sense a person's discomfort and impatience and throw it back to them. After a very brief explanation of Benjamin, which may include indicating that he is autistic, I immediately sense an inward and an outward shift in the person's attitude. Most people are extremely willing to make special accommodations for Benjamin. We have successfully called ahead to restaurants to place Benjamin's food order so that he has something to focus on immediately upon arriving at a restaurant. We have requested outdoor seating when Benjamin has become agitated inside a restaurant.

I think it is also important for people to know that autistic children have lots of different characteristics, just like the general population. Dustin Hoffman's portrayal of an autistic adult in the movie *Rain Man* served to bring the condition into mainstream awareness, but it has also had the effect of limiting what the public thinks when they hear the word "autistic." I believe that it is important for people to see autistic children, so that they know there is nothing to fear. If there is less fear about the condition, there will be more and more opportunities for our autistic children as they age.

Learn to trust your intuition, and refuse to be ruled by fear. Whenever you are making a decision about your child's health, ask yourself if you are doing it out of fear or because you feel that it will be an effective treatment for your child.

Become the most learned authority on your child's condition. Don't surrender your power to a physician or any one therapist. Educate yourself on therapies that seem to work. In my opinion, the two most important resources for any parent of an autistic child are Stephanie Marohn's *The Natural Medicine Guide to Autism* and Dr. Stephanie Cave's *What Your Doctor May Not Tell You About Children's Vaccinations*. Stephanie Marohn, a medical journalist, outlines 14 natural medicine treatment options for autistic children. I have successfully used many of these treatments. All of the treatments emphasize the goal of attaining the highest level of health for your child, not just a decrease in autistic symptoms.

Although I credit LEAP therapy for much of Benjamin's improvement, I believe that there are many ways to achieve whole body health in these children. In Stephanie Marohn's book, she details Dr. Dietrich Klinghardt's paradigm of body-mind-spirit healing, which includes electromagnetic balancing. One method for achieving this is NAET (Nambudripad's Allergy Elimination Techniques), which is based on acupuncture and works on the energy pathways of the meridians to eliminate the allergies that are so common in these children. This therapy seems very similar to the combinations of therapies we used with Benjamin.

Read accounts written by autistic adults. Donna Williams's book *Nobody Nowhere* provided invaluable insight on Benjamin's perception of the world. Children today should benefit from the experiences of others and not be forced to repeat them. Consider trying the dairy/gluten-free, low salicylate, additive-free diet that has worked so well for Donna Williams and for Benjamin. This is an inexpensive and relatively simple method of determining whether there are gut function issues affecting your child. This diet, along with the daily L-glutamine supplement, provided the greatest benefits to Benjamin for the least amount of time and resources invested.

Use your intuition when deciding on therapies for your child. Use your intuition coupled with scientific knowledge when deciding how and when to immunize your children. In *What Your Doctor May Not Tell You About Children's Vaccinations,* Dr. Cave offers some good common-sense advice about when to do this and why. If your child is sensitive to medications, just be aware that when your child becomes ill, there are effective alternative treatments that do not involve introducing chemical substances into the body.

This is our very personal story and my own interpretations of my son's condition as I have observed it. Since a diagnosis of an autism spectrum disorder is a "catchall" diagnosis, I believe that there is great diversity in the abilities and characteristics of these children. In fact, even among adults who are considered autistic there are vast differences. Temple Grandin describes herself as an extremely visual thinker and has written widely about thinking in pictures. She finds words easy to translate directly into mental pictures. Donna Williams describes herself as a visual learner, but perceives through movement, form, and feel. If there is no movement or a concept possesses no physical form, then its meaning is lost on her. Words alone do not create any pictures for her.

There are great strengths and abilities in other children that Benjamin does not appear to possess. This is the beauty of individuality. My hope is that each parent or caregiver reclaims the power over their child's condition and discerns for themselves what is appropriate for increasing the comfort level of the individual child and what abilities and traits should be encouraged and supported. May you have all the love, support, and encouragement to accomplish this goal.

Toilet Training Protocol

This approach to toilet training by Janet Boutton, Benjamin's first teacher, is based on the principles of positive reinforcement and positive practice. Simply put, we are helping the child make the connection that it is a *good* thing to be dry by using *positive reinforcement*. And when there is an accident, *positive practice teaches* the child that the "pee" (or whatever term you choose to use) goes in the toilet. Here are the guidelines and procedures to follow:

• The child wears underwear—no more diapers!

• Push fluids all day long.

• Dry pants check *every 5 minutes*. When doing this, take the child's hand and have them directly touch the underwear, then say, "You are dry—good job!" Then give the child a tangible reinforcer that has been chosen for the individual child.

• Every 30 minutes, sit the child on the toilet for several (about 5) minutes and wait for them to void in the toilet. Have fun things in the toilet area to keep the child occupied and to give them the idea that sitting on the toilet is a desired thing. If the child voids in the toilet, then you have a "potty party"—lots of social praise and some powerful reinforcer that has been chosen exclusively for the child's "potty party." If the child does not void during this time, get up and continue the dry pants checks every 5 minutes and the intervals of sitting on the toilet every 30 minutes.

• *If there is an accident:* Take the child by the hand and walk them quickly to the toilet *from the site of the accident,* saying very positively but neutrally (not in a scolding tone), "Pee goes in the potty." When you get to the toilet, take the child's pants down, sit them on the toilet for about 5 seconds, again saying, "Pee goes in the toilet." Take the child off the toilet, pull up the pants, and return to the site of the accident. Repeat this procedure five times. (Note: After the first few accidents, I found that repeating this procedure once or twice was sufficient.)

• After the child is changed, begin the dry pants checks and the sitting on the toilet every 30 minutes once again.

• Having the child clean up the accident is *NOT* part of this toilet training procedure.

This protocol should *not* be used with children who have moderate to severe involuntary avoidance diversion retaliation responses due to chronic fight-flight exposure anxiety. Because these children interpret praise and encouragement as a social invasion, this protocol could serve to inhibit toilet training in these children.

The following steps should be reviewed before beginning the protocol:

Step 1: Obtain a baseline measure with regard to your child's toileting behavior at home and at school. A simple baseline measure may provide updated objective information about the specific times that the child may urinate or defecate, whether it is in the potty, in pull-ups, or in his clothing.

Step 2: The toilet training program should be prioritized as the educational focus for a reasonable period of time. At school, the toilet training program should be one of, if not *the,* major educational priority for the child.

Step 3: The child will be best toilet-trained if he wears under-pants instead of pull-ups or diapers.

Step 4: The toileting schedule should be implemented consistently across the school and home settings, and should ideally be developed according to the baseline data collection.

At home and school, the adults working with the child may use a type of stopwatch that can be worn around the neck. The stopwatch can be set at any interval of time and then it beeps at that point in time. This allows a person to maintain a consistent toileting schedule even when busy with other activities.

Step 5: While toilet training, provide the child with extra fluids during the day.

Step 6: During times when the child is sitting on the potty, the adults in both the home and school should provide him with a highly reinforcing object. Pick an object that is very important to or highly desired by the child, such as a small battery-operated handheld fan, a Game Boy, or a favorite book.

The child's access to this object should be restricted so that the child is able to receive the object only when he is sitting on the potty. He should specifically not have access to this object at any other time during the initial phase of the toileting program. All adults should remember that the object will be initially provided simply based upon the toileting schedule and that receiving this object is not contingent upon the child actually urinating or defecating in the potty.

Step 7: When the child does urinate or defecate in the potty, adults should use ample social praise in order to build up and reinforce the appropriate toileting behavior. Adults should use whatever terms are meaningful to the child in regard to social attention and approval from adults.

Step 8: If the child should have an accident in his clothing, the adult working with him should refrain from any scolding or verbal criticism. It is worthwhile to try to label the incorrect response to the child as long as it is not done in a harsh or punitive manner. The adult should use a very neutral approach while still labeling the undesired behavior by saying the child's name, then "no wet pants, no dirty pants."

Step 9: When helping the child during times when he needs to be cleaned or changed, the adult should also handle this situation in as neutral a manner as possible. The idea here is not to be punitive, but instead, the goal is not to provide attention during the time that his clothing is being changed.

Benjamin's Charts

Good Behavior
Laughing
Playing
Sitting down
Sitting quietly
Hugging
Talking
Playing with toys

Bad Behavior
Fussing
Whining
Crying
Kicking
Screaming
Opening/shutting
  drawers/doors

Dressing
Benjamin sleeping
Benjamin ready to get dressed
  (in pajamas)
Pull pants down
Pull pull-ups down
Take shirt off
Throw pajamas in hamper
Underwear on
Socks on
Pants on
Pull pants up
Shirt on
Shoes on
Brush hair
Brush teeth
Put sunscreen on

Riding the Train

Waiting for the train
Waiting behind the yellow line
Boarding the train
Riding the train
Watching the big train go by
Eating ice cream
Walking down the street
Looking at the cookies in the
    bakery
See the musical instruments
Walking back to the train
Boarding the train
Riding the train
Walking home

Airplane Trip

Arriving at the airport terminal
Walking to the gate
Waiting at the gate
Walking onto the plane
Sitting in the seat
Playing with toys
Reading books
Eating snacks
Flight attendants serving bever-
    ages and snacks
Drinking juice
Listening to tapes
Arriving at airport
Traveling to final destination

Endnotes

Introduction

1. *A Parent's Tears,* reprinted with permission of Southwest Autism Research Center, 5040 East Shea Blvd., #166, Scottsdale, AZ 85254. After a diligent search, we were unable to locate the author. If the author will contact the publisher, we will be happy to credit the author in subsequent printings.

2. Clarissa Pinkola Estes, *Women Who Run with the Wolves* (New York: Ballantine, 1996), pp. 216–219. Cited in Elizabeth Harper Neeld, *A Sacred Primer: The Essential Guide to Quiet Time and Prayer,* p. 74.

Chapter 3

1. Dr. David Baskin, "Testimony to the Congressional Oversight Committee on Government Reform," December 10, 2002; available on the Internet at www.reform.house.gov/WHR.

2. Ibid.

3. Reprinted with permission from the American Psychiatric Association, *Statistical Manual of Mental Disorders,* Fourth Edition (Washington, DC: APA, 1994), pp. 70–71.

4. Ibid., pp. 67, 69.

5. Patricia M. Rodier, *The Early Origins of Autism: A Scientific American Article* (iBooks ISBN B00006BNPL, 2000), pp. 56–63.

6. Stanley Greenspan, M.D., Barry Prizant, Ph.D., and Amy Wetherby, Ph.D., "Is Your Baby Meeting These Important Milestones? Key Social, Emotional, and Communication Milestones for Your Baby's Healthy Development," First Signs, 2001. For developmental milestones from 4 months to 3 years; available on the

Internet at: http://www.firstsigns.org/pages/healthy_development/milestones. html.

7. "The Work of Byron Katie"; for a form of self-inquiry that can radically change the way you look at problems, see http://www.thework.org/intro.html.

8. Quote by Chuck Gardner, in "State Aid Sought for Autism" by Jennifer Coleman, *San Jose Mercury News* (November 24, 2002).

Chapter 4

1. Stephen M. Edelson, Ph.D., "Stereotypic (Self-Stimulatory) Behavior," Center for the Study of Autism, Salem, Oregon; see http://www.autism.org/stim.html.

2. Ibid.

3. Donna Williams, *Nobody Nowhere*, p. 10.

4. Ibid., p. 68.

Chapter 5

1. More detailed information on the therapy and a list of therapists can be obtained from The Upledger Institute, 11211 Prosperity Farms Road, Suite D-325, Palm Beach Gardens, FL 33410, tel: 561-622-4771, or by visiting their web site at www.upledger.com.

2. Stephanie Marohn, *The Natural Medicine Guide to Autism*, pp. 162-192.

3. Learning Enhancement Advanced Program (LEAP) developed by Dr. Charles T. Krebs, Ph.D., Melbourne Applied Physiology, 237 Rathdowne Street, Carlton, Victoria 3053, Australia.

4. Rosalyn L. Bruyere, *Wheels of Light*, p. 60.

5. Ibid., p. 61.

6. Ibid., p. 63.

7. From W. Brugh Joy, *Joy's Way*, pp. 30-31; reprinted by permission of Jeremy P. Tarcher, an imprint of Penguin Group (USA).

8. Ibid.

9. Valerie V. Hunt, *Infinite Mind*, pp. 19.

10. Ibid., p. 20.

11. Ibid.

12. Dietrich Klinghardt, M.D., Ph.D., quoted in Stephane Marohn, *The Natural Medicine Guide to Autism*, pp. 228-229.

13. Andrew J. Wakefield, "Testimony to the Congressional Oversight Committee on Government Reform," quoted in Stephanie Marohn, *The Natural Medicine Guide to Autism*, pp. 46-47; available on the Internet at www.house.gov/reform/ hearings/healthcare/01.04.25/wakefield.htm.

14. Stephanie Cave, *What Your Doctor May Not Tell You About Children's Vaccinations*, p. 39.

15. Ibid., pp. 61-62.

16. Dr. David Baskin, "Testimony to the Congressional Oversight Committee on Government Reform," December 10, 2002, available on the Internet at www.house.gov/reform.

17. Tim O'Shea, D.C., "Autism and Mercury: The San Diego Conference," report on the DAN! 2000 Conference, September 15, 2000, San Diego, California. Quoted in Stephanie Marohn, *The Natural Medicine Guide to Autism*, p. 46.

18. Stephanie Cave, *What Your Doctor May Not Tell You About Children's Vaccinations,* pp. 63–64; also see Stephanie Marohn, *The Natural Medicine Guide to Autism,* pp. 58–59.

19. Stephanie Cave, *What Your Doctor May Not Tell You About Children's Vaccinations,* pp. 107–113.

20. Ibid., p. 113.

21. See the Upledger Institute, at www.upledger.com/therapies/ltd.htm.

22. Donna Eden, *Energy Medicine,* p. 47.

23. Valerie V. Hunt, *Infinite Mind,* pp. 71-72.

24. Donna Williams's web site is www.donnawilliams.net. I found her Personal page and Autism Information page, particularly the Dietary Intervention and Autism, Savant Syndrome, Autism and Art, and "Waking Up Stories" pages very informative. All of Donna's eight books are available through her web site.

25. Donna Williams explains secretory IgA functions: "IgA is an immunoglobulin, an immune system messenger, that serves as a kind of flag to tell other parts of the body what to do and where to do it. It exists in the blood as serum IgA and in some people these levels in the blood can be normal even though another type of IgA, secretory IgA, may be insufficient or even completely absent. Secretory IgA is the body's first line of immune defense and lines the mucous membranes of the ears, nose, throat, lungs and digestive tract. The test for secretory IgA is not a blood test such as that for serum IgA, but a simple saliva swab. One of the main functions of secretory IgA in the mucous membranes of the gut is to put up a flag, so to speak, to signal organs like the pancreas and liver to release specific digestive enzymes required to properly digest the specific proteins it has identified as entering the digestive tract as food. It also puts up a flag to the fighter cells in the body to come and fight infections in the ears, nose, throat, lungs and gut. Without the flag, there are no enzymes and without the flag, the fighter cells don't arrive or if they are present they sit there like sitting ducks waiting to be infected. People with little or no secretory IgA cannot fight their own candida and often will carry other viral and bacterial infections in the gut which weigh down their resources. As candida takes over the gut, leaky gut develops and undigested foods, as well as harmful gut bacteria, can enter into the bloodstream and general circulation in the body. With little or no secretory IgA, mycoplasma, the tiny bacteria which exists in the air and settles on the food we eat, meets little or no defense in the mucous membranes of the ears, nose, throat, lungs and gut of these people. When a person develops leaky gut, these mycoplasma can enter the bloodstream, crusting up the surface of blood cells, infecting white cells which cripples the immune system and greatly impairs the ability of red blood cells to transport oxygen, and other nutrients around the body. The suppressed immune system leads to an inflammatory state throughout the body and the blood brain barrier itself can become inflamed. Infections and undigested proteins may then directly affect the brain, triggering neurotransmitter imbalances that underlie a range of autism related problems."

26. For a low salicylates, food additive-free diet see www.everybody.co.nz/docsq_w/salicylt.htm and www.fedupwithfoodadditives.info/, *Fed Up* and *The Failsafe Cookbook* by Sue Dengate. We used only the dairy and gluten-free recipes.

27. For information on Dr. Edward Danczak's biochemical approach to autism, see www.autismmanagement.com. The web site contains a helpful model for relationships among alternative approaches to autism spectrum disorders and explanations of each step of the treatment protocol.

28. Developed by Peggy Phoenix Dubro; for additional information, see www.emfbalancingtechnique.com.

Chapter 6

1. Donna Williams, *Nobody Nowhere,* p. 201.

Chapter 7

1. A term coined by Leo Kanner, John Hopkins psychiatrist and autism pioneer, to refer to the advanced skill areas of autistic children.

2. Donna Eden, *Energy Medicine,* p. 17.

3. Ibid., p. 43.

4. *DreamHealer: His Name is Adam,* book available via www.dreamhealer.com and www.hrpub.com.

5. Valerie V. Hunt, *Infinite Mind,* p. 143.

6. Roger Nelson, Director, Global Consciousness Project, "Terrorist Disaster, September 11, 2001," p. 1; see http://noosphere.princeton.edu.

Chapter 8

1. Valerie V. Hunt, *Infinite Mind,* p. 76.

2. Ibid., p. 26.

3. Ibid., pp. 246–247.

Chapter 9

1. Barbara Harris Whitfield, *Spiritual Awakenings,* p. 89.

2. Leonard Shlain, *The Alphabet Versus the Goddess,* pp. 18, 19.

3. Ibid., pp. 19–20, 21.

4. Barbara Harris Whitfield, *Spiritual Awakenings,* pp. 92–93.

5. Ibid., p. 90.

6. Madeleine Nash, "The Secrets of Autism," *Time* (April 29, 2002).

7. Donna Williams, *Nobody Nowhere,* p. 71.

8. Ibid., pp. 70–71.

9. Ibid., p. 133.

10. Leonard Shlain, *The Alphabet Versus the Goddess,* pp. 24–25.

11. Valerie V. Hunt, *Infinite Mind,* p. 111.

12. Ibid.

13. Ibid., p. 112.

14. Donna Williams, *Nobody Nowhere,* p. 138.

15. Ibid., p. 70.

16. Sandra Blakeslee, "A Boy, a Mother, and a Rare Map of Autism's World," *New York Times* (November 19, 2002).

17. Valerie V. Hunt, *Infinite Mind,* p. 83.

18. Ibid.

19. Ibid.

20. Ibid., pp. 93–94.

21. Ibid., p. 94.

22. Ibid., pp. 109–110.

23. Ibid., p. 77.

24. John J. Falone, *The Genius Frequency*, pp. 258–259.

25. Donna Williams, *Nobody Nowhere*, pp. 201–202.

Chapter 11

1. Donna Williams, *Nobody Nowhere*, p. 43.

2. Ibid., p. 48.

3. John Taylor Gatto, "A Short Angry History of American Forced Schooling," a speech delivered to the Vermont Homeschoolers Conference; see http://members.11.net/chiliast/pdocs/education/angry_history.htm.

Chapter 12

1. F. David Peat, "Synchronicity: Bridge Between Matter and Mind," p. 1; see www.fdavidpeat.com.

2. F. David Peat, "Time, Synchronicity and Evolution," p. 1; see www.fdavid-peat.com.

3. F. David Peat, "Synchronicity: Bridge Between Matter and Mind," p. 1.

4. F. David Peat, "The Speculum of Inscape and Landscape," p. 1; see www.fdavidpeat.com.

5. Ibid., p. 3.

6. F. David Peat, "Synchronicity: Bridge Between Matter and Mind," p. 1.

7. Barbara Harris Whitfield, *Spiritual Awakenings*, p. 127.

Chapter 14

1. Donna Williams, *Nobody Nowhere*, pp. 83–84

2. Ibid., pp. 79–80.

3. Ibid., p. 206.

4. Kahlil Gibran, *The Prophet*, p. 56.

5. Ibid.

6. Donna Williams, *Nobody Nowhere*, p. 207.

Chapter 15

1. Sandra Blakeslee, "A Boy, a Mother, and a Rare Map of Autism's World," *New York Times* (November 19, 2002).

2. Kahlil Gibran, *The Prophet*, p. 56.

Chapter 16

1. Barbara Harris Whitfield, *Spiritual Awakenings*, p. 71.

2. John J. Falone, *The Genius Frequency*, p. 269.

3. Ibid.

4. Valerie V. Hunt, *Infinite Mind,* p. 70.

5. Barbara Harris Whitfield, *Spiritual Awakenings,* p. 71.

6. For additional information on Leap toys, see their web site at www.leapfrogtoys.com.

7. For additional information on the Wiggles, see their web site at www.thewiggles.com. For video ordering information in the U.S., see http://store.yahoo.com/lyrickstudios/wiggles.html.

8. *I Love Toy Trains—The Music Video,* TM Books & Video, Box 279, New Buffalo, MI 49117, tel: 800-892-2822, www.tmbooks-video.com.

9. Kathi Appelt, *The Alley Cat's Meow* (San Diego, California: Harcourt, 2002).

10. Valerie V. Hunt, *Infinite Mind,* p. 143.

11. Ibid., p. 110.

12. Stephanie Marohn, *The Natural Medicine Guide to Autism,* p. 84.

13. Benjamin Iobst, *Seven Metals, Singing Bowls of Tibet.* Ordering information is Compact Disc, P.O. Box 61, Orefield, PA 18069-0061.

14. *Macaroni Pony,* limited availability through Monroe Products, P.O. Box 505, Lovingston, VA 22949, tel: 434-263-8692, Interstate@Hemi-Sync.com, www.hemi-sync.com.

15. *Robbie the Rabbit,* produced by Monroe Products, P.O. Box 505, Lovingston, VA 22949, tel: 434-263-8692, www.hemi-sync.com.

16. *Joy Jumper,* produced by Monroe Products, P.O. Box 505, Lovingston, VA 22949, tel: 434-263-8692, www.hemi-sync.com.

17. Barbara Harris Whitfield, *Spiritual Awakenings,* p. 108.

18. Ibid., p. 110.

19. Ibid.

Bibliography

Bruyere, Rosalyn L. *Wheels of Light: Chakras, Auras, and the Healing Energy of the Body.* New York: Fireside, 1994.

Cave, Stephanie. *What Your Doctor May Not Tell You About Children's Vaccinations.* New York: Warner Books, 2001.

Diagnostic and Statistical Manual of Mental Disorders, Fourth Edition. Washington, DC: American Psychiatric Association, 1994.

Eden, Donna. *Energy Medicine.* New York: Jeremy P. Tarcher, 1998.

Emoto, Masaru. *Messages from Water.* Tokyo: HADO Kyoikusha, 2001

Falone, John J. *The Genius Fequency: An Owner's Manual for the Cosmic Mind.* e-book experience, DivineArts, www.thegeniusfrequency.com.

Gibran, Kahlil, *The Prophet.* New York: Random House, 2001.

Hay, Louise L. *You Can Heal Your Life.* Carlsbad, California: Hay House, 1999.

Hunt, Valerie V. *Infinite Mind: Science of the Human Vibrations of Consciousness.* Malibu, California: Malibu Publishing, 1996.

Joy, W. Brugh. *Joy's Way: A Map for the Transformational Journey.* New York: Jeremy P. Tarcher, 1979.

Marohn, Stephanie. *The Natural Medicine Guide to Autism.* Charlottesville, Virginia: Hampton Roads, 2002.

Neeld, Elizabeth Harper. *A Sacred Primer: The Essential Guide to Quiet Time and Prayer.* Los Angeles: Renaissance Books, 1999.

Seroussi, Karyn. *Unraveling the Mystery of Autism and Pervasive Developmental Disorder: A Mother's Story of Research and Recovery.* New York: Broadway Books, 2002.

Shlain, Leonard. *The Alphabet Versus the Goddess: The Conflict Between Word and Image.* New York: Viking, 1998.

Upledger, John E. *Your Inner Physician and You: CranioSacral Therapy and SomatoEmotional Release.* Berkeley, California: North Atlantic Books, 1997.

Whitfield, Barbara Harris. *Spritual Awakenings: Insights of the Near-Death Experience and Other Doorways to Our Soul.* Deerfield Beach, Florida: Health Communications, 1995.

Williams, Donna. *Nobody Nowhere: The Extraordinary Autobiography of an Autistic.* New York: Times Books, 1992.

About the Author

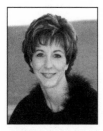 Keli Lindelien was born in Mission, Texas, and spent her childhood in the Rio Grande Valley area of South Texas. She attended Texas A&M University in College Station, Texas, earning a B.B.A. in marketing. After working for several years, and volunteering at a legal aid society, she decided to attend law school, earning a J.D. from South Texas College of Law in Houston, Texas. She worked as a family law attorney, and after her daughter was born she worked part-time as a juvenile prosecutor. She served on the board of directors of a child advocacy center and as assistant director and assistant to the director of the George Bush Presidential Library Foundation until the demands of her son's condition took priority over her professional career, and she began working on the most intriguing case of her life.

She and her family currently reside in South Australia.

Hampton Roads Publishing Company

. . . for the evolving human spirit

Hampton Roads Publishing Company
publishes books on a variety of subjects,
including metaphysics, health,
visionary fiction, and other related topics.

For a copy of our latest catalog, call toll-free
(800) 766-8009, or send your name and address to:

Hampton Roads Publishing Company, Inc.
1125 Stoney Ridge Road
Charlottesville, VA 22902

e-mail: hrpc@hrpub.com
www.hrpub.com